Shift from
to Inter

Amaging™
GROWING OLD ON PURPOSE

Margie Hackbarth

© 2021 Amaging, LLC
All rights reserved.

No part of this publication in print or in electronic format may be reproduced, stored in a retrieval system, or transmitted in any form or by any means, electronic, mechanical, photocopying, recording, or otherwise without the prior written permission of the publisher.

The scanning, uploading, and distribution of this book without permission is a theft of the author's intellectual property. If you would like permission to use material from the book (other than for review purposes), please contact amaging.info@gmail.com. Thank you for your support of the author's rights.

Distribution by Bublish, Inc.

ISBN: 978-1-647043-52-0 (hardback)
ISBN: 978-1-647043-51-3 (paperback)
ISBN: 978-1-647043-50-6 (eBook)

To my circle of loving family and friends
who model and share your *Amaging*-ness™.
I appreciate each of you.

Special thanks to editors
Phil Ransom and Dick Sine

THANK YOU

Thank you for reading *Amaging*™ **Growing Old On Purpose**.

Amaging™ is a term I coined that rhymes with *amazing*. It means to cause great surprise or wonder later in life. It describes astonishing or startlingly impressive accomplishments while aging.

I invite you to visit www.amaging.info for updates and free resources.

Your feedback regarding this book will be welcomed and appreciated.

—Margie Hackbarth, Author

Contents

1. *Amaging*™ Growing Old On Purpose 1
2. The Power of Words and Affirmations 13
3. Why Do You Want It? 31
4. Become More Aware of Age Bias 39
5. More Than Fluff 51
6. Setting *Amaging*™ Goals as We Age 59
7. Thinking with the Enemy 71
8. New Tricks for "Old Dogs" 79
9. Having Good Friends and Being a Good Friend 91
10. Better Fitness While Growing Old 105
11. Better Food Habits While Growing Old 117
12. Strengthening Our Faith While Growing Old 129
13. The Pain Is Real and So Is the Fatigue 143
14. Practice Makes Better 147
15. End on a High Note 157

Appendix 1: *Amaging*™ Affirmation and Action Plan 165
Works Cited 167
Table of Affirmations 175

1

Amaging™
Growing Old On Purpose

Remember the popular children's story about a railroad superintendent who wanted a strong engine to pull a heavy train up a big hill? As the story goes, some of the bigger engines in his yard declined for reasons they thought were very good. They had been up and down those tracks before, so many times before. The train was too heavy. The hill too steep—or so they thought. The superintendent asked a smaller locomotive to do the job, and the brave, little engine said, "I think I can." Then, as the little train's challenging journey chugged along, it repeated its mantra, "I think I can, I think I can," until it successfully reached the summit and said, "I can!"

This little engine put out a simple message: when you face what might seem like an impossible task, if you focus on the positive, you can do more than you first thought. It's not surprising that this little engine story has withstood the test of time. It's an original work by Rev. Charles S. Wing, who first told the story in a sermon to his congregation in Brooklyn, New York, and his sermon was later published in the *New York Times* in 1906. Watty Piper, under the pen name of Arnold Munk, retold the story in 1957 in the illustrated children's book, *The*

Little Engine That Could (Piper, 1957). The children's book enjoyed popularity for decades, and in 2017 it was even turned into a musical with an emphasis on perseverance (Wichmann, 2017).

Although the story became popular as a children's book, this inspiring sermon was first intended for people of all ages. Rev. Wing shared it with his congregation of old and young. Many older adults, myself included, fully bought into his "I think I can" message as a child. Yet, somewhere along life's journey, we began to doubt ourselves. "I think I can" turned into "I might be able to" or "I'll see what I can do" or "I'm not sure I'm up for it," and later into even less affirming self-talk. And just like that, we found ourselves thinking self-limiting thoughts.

Do any of the following ring true for you?

> *Dancing is for young people.*
> *I just can't do this anymore!*
> *I don't have the energy to learn a new trade.*
> *I did my part.*
> *Why bother? I won't be able to do it anyway.*
> *She/he is so smart. I'll never be as smart as her/him.*
> *I'm too set in my ways to learn new _____ (fill in the blank).*
> *_____ (fill in the blank) is for younger people.*

Older adults have seen a lot, heard a lot, and felt a lot, and while we may forget more recent experiences, we often remember the long-term lessons learned. We generally remember our fears, things that may have embarrassed us, past mistakes, or failures. For many people, as more years are lived, a can-do attitude unintentionally morphs into something closer to an uninterested spirit.

Sound familiar? This common mindset shift may begin much earlier than we realize. Researchers have found that the tendency to be less open to new things will increase for most people as early as the third decade of life (Westerhoff, December 2008).

While this tendency is disheartening, there's good reason to be optimistic. Look around your family, your circle of friends, and your community. You can likely name older adults who buck this trend, do amazing (or *amaging*™ things), and cultivate a can-do spirit. Perhaps they are retired accountants helping low-income people file their taxes, gainfully employed sixty-somethings surpassing sales quotas, volunteers driving disabled people to medical appointments, dedicated elder church members helping refugees settle in a new land, talented seamstresses making warm clothing and quilts for those less fortunate, highly literate professionals leading community book clubs, or well-past-retirement hobbyists passing along their skill sets to a younger generation. One such individual I will introduce you to later in this chapter is Ginny, a kind, hardworking, and God-fearing grandmother. The list goes on.

I coined the word *amaging*™ as an expression to encourage older adults to do amazing things.

Here's my working definition of *amaging*™ (rhymes with "amazing"):
1. Causing great surprise or wonder later in life
2. Astonishing or startlingly impressive accomplishments while aging

---

This book focuses on the *amaging*™ possibilities within all of us, the use of affirmations to support our goals while growing older, and the need for affirmations to help offset our aging-opposed culture. Affirmations are words declaring something positive and helpful in a way that will bring about positive changes.

When we look, we find *amaging*™ individuals everywhere. Anyone can become *amaging*.™ While reading this book, consider ways you might rekindle an "I think I can" spirit and make the most of each day remaining in this part of life's journey. Consider the ways you shift from reluctantly aging to intentionally aging. Throughout this book, I share a framework for affirmations to help older adults counter some of the negative stereotypes associated with aging. I call this framework, "*Amaging™ Affirmations.*" The first six chapters of this book build a foundation for this framework and explain more about what an affirmation is and how it is used, and why words are powerful.

Chapter 7 is devoted entirely to rethinking how we talk to ourselves without "Thinking with the Enemy." On my bookshelf, I have a fun book of lists, *Lists to Live By* (Gray, 2001, Second Collection), and it includes these tips for growing older:

> *Your humor is not over; enjoy it.*
> *Your strength is not gone; use it.*
> *Your opportunities have not vanished; pursue them.*
> *God is not dead; seek Him.*

I love this "list to age by" so to speak. Each of the items relates to a "don't give up" mindset or, rather, a growth mindset, not a fixed mindset.

Both growth and fixed mindsets are differentiated in a popular book, *Mindset,* by Carol Dweck (Dweck, 2007). Mindsets guide how we interpret the happenings around us. According to Dweck, a person with a growth mindset embraces challenges, is persistent, learns from other people's feedback, sees effort as a way to master something, and is inspired by successful people. A growth mindset helps confront a shortcoming, while a fixed mindset finds it easier (and perhaps just fine) to live in a world without shortcomings! A growth mindset seeks challenge and even thrives on those challenges—stretching and growing because of them. Not surprisingly, Dweck asserts that we are all born with a growth mindset, and while this may shift toward fixed over time (or in different situations), people can use a growth mindset to help get past setbacks.

People with a fixed mindset don't take failure well, because they believe they shouldn't fail at all. A fixed mindset makes your ego hurt when you fail because you feel you already know it all. On the contrary, a growth mindset adapts to failure. A growth mindset helps you open your mind to learn more.

Much of Dweck's material helps students learn and do better in the classroom, as well as helps people who face negative stereotypes, such as underserved populations and females (Mahmud, 2017). I would advocate that a growth mindset is important for older adults who either knowingly or unknowingly encounter age bias. I'll discuss the negative age stereotype further in chapter four, and growth mindsets are explored in the *Amaging™ Affirmations* throughout this book.

In the *amaging™* framework for affirmations, pausing to consider your mindset is an important step: What is your growth mindset to support this? Mindset matters because changes begin with the brain, and then behaviors follow. Habits are behaviors. Habits include routines, practices, and customs that have become part of our life. Sometimes, as older adults, we think we are too "set in our ways" to acquire a new habit, or more importantly, to replace a not-so-good habit with a better one. Not true! New habits can be learned at any age. Acquiring new habits has less to do with age and more to do with mindset.

In addition to mindset, the framework for affirmations asks you to consider what new "hats" you may need to wear. What do hats have to do with growing older? The answer doesn't relate to warm ears or a warm head. As older adults looking back on our lives, we may recall times when we were required to "wear a new hat" or "wear multiple hats." This is an idiom used when we have more than one task or duty to perform, more than one role to perform at one time.

Sometimes, we have had to take on one or more new roles in order to get the job done. For example, early on in my career I worked for a small community hospital and I wore many hats, with community relations responsibilities for not only marketing but also for fundraising and volunteer coordination. A stay-at-home mom may wear different hats as the family's housekeeper, cook, tutor, chauffeur, nurse, and bookkeeper. An empty nester may wear different hats as a traveler, community volunteer, hobbyist, and caregiver for an aging parent or a young grandchild. Throughout this book, consider what new hats you may want to try on and wear as you grow older. It's likely you have created an identity you are proud of—or should be proud of. As you set and achieve new goals, there is no need to produce an entirely new identity. Put on a new hat from time to time—it can help you master something new.

In chapters 9 to 12, you'll find specific examples of *Amaging*™ *Affirmations* applied to important healthy aging concerns:

- Loneliness (chapter 9)
- Fitness (chapter 10)
- Nutrition (chapter 11)
- Faith and Spirituality (chapter 12).

I identified these topics as concerns for older adults while I performed the research for this book. I also culled them from my interactions with older adults and my experience working with health-care organizations.

At What Age Are We "Old"?

This book is written for those who self-identify as an older adult and have had the privilege of growing old. I am often asked, "At what age is someone 'old'?" When I worked as a service line administrator for a senior health service line, I was frequently asked about the ages of my target audience. I was also asked about when a person falls into the "senior" category.

In the United States, a geriatrician or physician who specializes in the care of older adults may want to begin seeing a patient at the age of sixty-five for an initial "Welcome to Medicare" visit. Thereafter, this doctor will want to see the patient yearly for a wellness visit and as needed for injuries or illnesses. A geriatrician may consider ages 65 to 75 as "young-old," 75 to 85 as "old," and 85 and beyond as "old-old."

A clinical nurse educator once told me that aging begins in our early twenties and, once puberty ends, our bodies begin a gradual transition toward aging. How gradual this transition will be over time varies for each of us. I don't advocate that we are "old" soon after puberty, and I don't advocate that becoming "old" begins during our "Welcome to Medicare" visit. The actual year or years we transition into growing old are based on many factors. For some, a "growing old" feeling may begin during the decade leading into retirement. For others, it begins at the onset of retirement. For some, it begins well past retirement, after new routines or social circles are formed. For many, the "growing old" feeling is never fixed—it ebbs and flows depending upon health, physical function, socialization, and other factors.

With this book, I want to avoid slotting people into a category based on age, and help people overcome feeling stuck due to more years lived. I'm recommending a framework for affirmations to help older adults do amazing things—be more *amaging*™! This framework, described in chapter two, is a point of reference—similar to a compass—that guides and moves you forward. When used in its entirety, I refer to this framework as an *Amaging*™ *Affirmation*. Like the little engine, your joints, brain speed, strength, and physical function may not be where they were in your earlier years, or you may think they fall short.

Throughout this book, you'll find many examples of *Amaging*™ *Affirmations*. The examples I have included relate to wellness habits and positive aging, such as becoming more physically active, eating less sugar, reducing portion sizes, fostering friendships, improving a prayer habit, and more. You will also find step-by-step instructions to help you create your own *Amaging*™ *Affirmations* to keep you chugging forward, enjoying the journey with *amaging*™ momentum.

About Self-Efficacy

Setting and achieving small goals are an important element of "chugging forward." As older adults, when we are successful and achieve small wins, we build our self-efficacy—our confidence in our ability to do things. Self-efficacy is a theory originated by Albert Bandura, and it is defined as "an optimistic self-belief in our competence or chances of successfully accomplishing a task and producing a favorable outcome." Bandura asserts that self-efficacy is a type of confidence, and that it can come from mastering past experiences, observing role models who do well, being persuaded of our capability by an influential person, having a positive emotional state (i.e., not depressed or stressed), and using our own imagination (Maddux, 2005).

By setting small, daily goals, older adults can improve their lives. Bandura asserts that past experiences top the list of components of self-efficacy; after that, we can build experience through small, daily goals that gradually build self-efficacy for wellness management as a whole (PositivePsychology.org.uk, 2008). Sadly, older adults report lower self-efficacy than middle-aged and younger adults when it comes to daily life decisions and health care (Woodward, 1987).

In a separate study, researchers found that low self-efficacy is linked to functional limitations, which are limitations in our day-to-day activities like walking, taking care of ourselves, climbing stairs, or lifting. During a study of 884 older adults, ages 65 to 88, researchers measured walking, way finding, time standing on one leg, and other activities, along with perceived functional limitations. They found evidence that self-efficacy was linked to physical function among the elders studied. The people in the study who could walk more often or walk further distances also had greater self-efficacy. The study concluded that test subjects with self-efficacy had fewer functional limitations; this was true regardless of whether they lived in a rural or urban environment (Mullen, 2012).

The framework for *Amaging*™ *Affirmations* described throughout this book can be used to help you achieve more goals, have more

wins, and gain self-efficacy. Think of the affirmation framework as your inner personal trainer who reboots your conviction to take more steps, reach your summit, and say, "I can, too!"

"If the Bus Is Going, I'm Going to Be on It!"

I had the pleasure of knowing an amazing woman who found an inner drive to live each day of her eighty-five years to the fullest. Her name was Ginny, and she volunteered at the hospital where I worked for a number of years in southwest Wisconsin. Ginny wasn't content to watch life from the sidelines. She wanted to be a part of the action, to jump into the middle and help make a difference regardless of what "game" was being played! In addition to caring for her family, Ginny volunteered for the local hospital's pie sale and quilt show, collected admission at the ballpark, worked in the 4-H malt stand, built parade floats, and helped in other ways as needed.

Ginny was a hard worker. When she was a hospital volunteer, there was no job Ginny was not willing to do. She often drove the car pool that collected other volunteers to help with special events. She also carried boxes of household items for a large-scale rummage sale in and out of a community building, browned pounds of ground beef for concession sloppy joes, and set up hundreds of quilt stands for a quilt show and then tore everything down and cleaned up afterward. These types of activities went on well into her retirement years, and these are just a few ways Ginny, along with her late husband, Donald, gave back to the small community that was their home for more than fifty years.

Ginny had earned a reputation as the "hostess with the mostest," and people enjoyed hanging out with her and attending her events. If Ginny was involved, there would be much laughter. I am challenged to remember specific jokes and punch lines, or I would share a few laughs I had with Ginny over the years. While researching this book, I talked with Ginny's grown daughter, who shared with me a story about Ginny distributing little gifts at a family gathering. She handed out a pair of disposable underwear for each woman in attendance! Apparently, these could be worn as panties and then put in the garbage. Always the practical one, Ginny suggested carrying them along in a suitcase on your next trip and then tossing them in the hotel garbage can.

I can picture Ginny buying these, wrapping them, and handing them out, all the while smiling to herself as she pictured the funny reactions she would get from the ladies. Ginny liked to find little things to brighten other people's days, and she often handed out small presents "just because." Ginny enjoyed hosting showers for new brides and new babies—my daughters included. I have a beautiful baby quilt packed away, God willing, to give to one of my own grandchildren someday. I'll happily pass along this treasured gift from a woman who was so special to me.

As was said to Ginny and her husband when they celebrated their sixtieth wedding anniversary, "Everyone was welcomed and made to feel important, loved, accepted, like they were a part of this family—the more the merrier!" This willingness to reach out and get involved continued even after Ginny and Donald moved into an assisted-living facility together. Her daughter told me that despite her mother's health challenges and painful struggle with osteoporosis, Ginny wanted to be active. The facility had an activities van to take residents out and about and to visit the local apple orchard, pick up groceries, take in a movie, and other excursions. Ginny once told her daughter, "If the bus is going, I'm going to be on it!" She didn't want to miss out on anything. Ever.

While Ginny had the confidence necessary to be active and enjoy new experiences—to "try on new hats," as I said at the start of this book—this confidence should not be confused with arrogance. Ginny was quite humble and oozed kindness, often repeating, "If you can't say something nice about someone, then don't say anything at all." These were not mere words for Ginny. Those who had the good fortune to know her saw how she lived by this motto throughout her life. She also had a gifted way of turning a negative conversation into a positive one. Ginny naturally looked for ways to defend and speak well of other people. I was truly blessed to know her.

In some ways, Ginny was one inspiration for this book. The world needs more people like Ginny, especially more older adults like her. The world needs more of her positive mindset, her willingness to befriend others, her energy, and her upbeat personality. While Ginny is probably an outlier in the normal bell curve of special people, there's no reason to think that those of us in the normal range can not move closer to Ginny's level of specialness! If we want to change something about ourselves, it's not too late. We can do it. Like the little engine going up a new and difficult hill, *thinking we can do it* can make the difference between achieving or not achieving new goals.

2

The Power of Words and Affirmations

> *Life's battles don't always go*
> *To the stronger or faster man;*
> *But sooner or later the man who wins*
> *Is the man who thinks he can.*
> (Walter Wintle, "The Man Who Thinks He Can")

Ask any Green Bay Packers football fan, "Why was the legendary coach Vince Lombardi so successful?" You'll learn that, in the hearts of Packers fans, Lombardi represents not only a winning coach but also a charismatic leader whose careful choice of words inspired a dejected team with a pathetic, losing record. In 1958, before Lombardi came on board, the team's record was dismal: they had just one win, ten losses, and one tie. Under Lombardi's leadership, the Packers rose to the top of their game, winning five NFL Championships and two Super Bowls.

Lombardi knew what it took for a team to become number one, and he found the words to make certain his players understood and acted accordingly. Lombardi influenced both his players and his fans with passionate stories and team speeches on topics such as commitment, mental toughness, habits, discipline, and getting results. A Packer fan base was born during Lombardi's years in Green Bay (1959 to 1967), with followers across Wisconsin and the nation falling in love with Lombardi, the Green and Gold, and the game of football.

Words can be powerful in much less extreme and sometimes lackluster situations! Sometimes, the power of words can be invisible to us. The curriculum for a chronic disease self-management workshop I've co-led includes discussion on healthy ways to "use your mind" as a tool to help manage some of the symptoms of an ongoing disease. Visual imagery is one tool within a "toolbox" of options to support self-management. One activity we do in each workshop involves asking participants to close their eyes and imagine holding a lemon. We don't pass around a basket of lemons—it's imaginary. Then participants imagine biting into the unpeeled lemon (gross, right?). It's not cut pieces of lemon, either; it's just biting into a whole lemon, peel and all.

Imagine how this would taste in your mouth and on your lips. What reactions are you feeling?

Some participants would say their lips would pucker, that they would salivate a little, and some would get a cringe feeling from biting into something very sour. The point to this story is that there was *not* a real lemon; yet most participants had some type of physical reaction when they imagined biting into one.

Try this yourself. What physical reactions do you feel? This lemon activity is an example of using words to imagine something that brings about a physical response. It shows that words can lead to physical responses.

ENTHUSIASM: LIKE AN OCEAN'S TIDE

Affirmations are words used to help spur a physical reaction and to help achieve goals. They also help to reinforce why you want that goal, who you are willing to become to get it, and what you're willing to do to get it. Vince Lombardi Jr. talks about his father's motivation in the best-selling book he co-authored with his father, Vince Lombardi Sr., *What It Takes to Be #1*. The younger author compared enthusiasm to "the tide in an ocean with a strong force to sweep obstacles away." As we think about little and large goals we might want to achieve, wouldn't it be great to have something as powerful as an ocean tide come through and sweep away the barriers that block our route to success?

Likely, it's easier to identify obstacles than it is to find ways to overcome them. Here are some common obstacles that I have encountered and that others have shared with me that prevent reaching goals:

- little time to work on a goal
- lack of consistent motivation
- resources, especially money
- pain, it physically hurts to work at it
- fear of associated problems that may arise when the goal is achieved

The list goes on. Affirmations can be used to bring about more consistent enthusiasm and help sweep away obstacles, similar to the enthusiasm Lombardi describes.

Affirmations are more fully defined later in this chapter. I will also introduce you to a framework for *Amaging™ Affirmations* that includes six steps to help you self-assess what you really want to accomplish along with the "why" behind it. It will also help you to reflect on what a growth mindset might be for someone who achieves this goal, as well as encourage you to identify a new hat you may need to wear (or type of person you are committed to become) and to detail the specific steps needed to make progress.

Most importantly, the framework includes encouragement and inspiration. An *Amaging™ Affirmation* isn't complete without considering what motivates you to move forward and make progress. Before we delve into this, I want to introduce the idea of strengths because you will want to lean on your strengths when you write your affirmations.

One way to help overcome the obstacles that crop up when you try to achieve a goal is to lean in on your personal character strengths. Examples of character strengths include things like bravery, perseverance, self-regulation, hope, spirituality, and so forth. The VIA Institute on Character Strengths (https://www.viacharacter.org/) has created an online survey to help people identify their character strengths. I have found this to be a valuable tool that I use to not only reflect on my positive qualities, but also to help me look for the positive qualities in others. VIA Institute has identified twenty-four character strengths, and we all have them to greater and lesser extents. When I took the assessment, I learned that some of my strengths include humor, forgiveness, curiosity, creativity, social intelligence, and humility. Some other strengths fell lower on my list. This doesn't mean I don't have them;—they are just lower on the list. My challenge is to lean on my top strengths to help me achieve my goals, to enjoy life, and to overcome struggles. I also look for ways to reflect on these strengths when I am discouraged.

When repeated often enough, character strength descriptions and other words found in *Amaging™ Affirmations* will become your thoughts. A favorite Pinterest board I have followed is a collection by Debbie Kay, founder of Hope for the Broken-Hearted Ministries. In one post Kay wrote, she hints at the value of affirmations: "The Bible says that as we think, so we are. If I want to be healed, whole, and full of joy and peace, I must take an active role in the process, take control of my thoughts." I would advocate that Kay shares great insight not only for the broken hearted, but also the happy or contented heart.

The Bible contains many affirmative phrases and references about the power of words. "Our words have the power to destroy and the power to build up" (Proverbs 12:6). Do you choose your words wisely to build up or tear down? To show kindness or cruelty? To complain or compliment? The words we use are not just the result of air coming from our lungs, past our vocal cords, and mixing with our tongue and lips to make sounds that form words. We can carefully choose what words are formed before the act of speech occurs. Choose wisely!

Affirmations are not intended to replace prayer, Bible study, or time spent in worship; however, the collection of affirmations included in this book can complement them and help reboot your energy to pray, study, or worship. Chapter 12 focuses on ways affirmations help strengthen faith. I've also included a list of Bible verses you may want to weave into your own affirmations.

It's important to repeat affirmations often, at least daily. Interestingly, Lombardi Jr. says that enthusiasm didn't come naturally for his father. It seems Coach Lombardi had to give himself a pep talk sometimes.

"Every day you've got to lay on some kindling, strike a match, and fan the flames of passion and zeal" (Lombardi, 2006).

Affirmations can become your own kindling, match, and personal fan to help ignite whatever it is you want to act upon!

Think of affirmations as an affordable and easy way to bring a Lombardi-like personal coach into your home on a daily basis—one who will light a fire under you and help you achieve your goals.

This book focuses on setting goals relating to things that matter most to many older adults, like making friendships, partaking in fitness activities, strengthening faith, and improving our diets. Later in the book, you will learn how to use affirmations like a morning and evening "tidal wave," to help sweep away any obstacles that are getting in the way of your important goals.

Amaging™ Affirmations

It's normal to question whether an affirmation can impact anything more physical than turning a frown into a smile. I was a skeptic, too. I am old school and think achievements come from behaviors like hard work, discipline, healthy living, and a strong prayer life, not by self-affirmation.

My opinion changed when I came to know Hal Elrod through his writings. Elrod is the author of *The Miracle Morning, Taking Life Head On, The Miracle Equation,* and several other books written as derivatives of *The Miracle Morning,* such as *The Miracle Morning for Writers,* which I found helpful while writing this book. Elrod shares what I believe is one of the best examples of the way an affirmation can influence a person's physical well-being in a dramatic way. Elrod was in a head-on car crash that left him with multiple injuries, including the loss of short-term memory from a traumatic brain injury. In his book, he tells the story of how he found himself repeatedly apologizing to others for his lack of recall. "I have a horrible memory," he would say. Over time this became his mantra. Seven years after his accident, he was still repeating it to himself and others—until he made a discovery. "Maybe my memory was horrible, in part, because I never made the effort to *think* I could improve it" (Elrod H., 2012).

This discovery led Elrod to write his first affirmation, encouraging himself to let go of his self-limiting mantra and to believe his brain's health and memory could improve. Over time, his memory gradually improved. From this, Elrod learned a powerful lesson: affirmations can help you improve many areas of your life. He looked for other ways to use affirmations to become more successful in life.

Are there any aspects of your life that you'd like to improve but have assumed it isn't possible? Imagine a goal you might want to set relating to physical fitness. Perhaps running a 5K? Or walking a 5K? Maybe your goal is just to walk around the block? Swim a lap? Swim a mile? Maneuver a kayak? Do chair yoga? Play pickleball?

Whatever type of physical exercise you would like to improve, it's important to make the effort to *think* you can improve before putting on tennis shoes, activewear, dance shoes, or a swimsuit. Just as Elrod found himself saying, "I have a horrible memory," there may be self-limiting messages you repeat to yourself or to others.

Here are a few examples of messages that may be preventing you from improving your physical fitness:

- I can't walk that far anymore.
- My exercise days are behind me.
- I never learned to swim, and I'm too old to learn now.
- Yoga is for young people.
- I am a klutz on the dance floor.
- I don't have the energy for _____ (fill in the blank).

Can you identify one of your own self-limiting thoughts from the above list, or a different thought of its kind? Take the first step toward achieving a new goal by affirming you can do it! Choose a growth mindset—positive and helpful, not fixed and limiting.

A few words of caution here. If you would like to set a new goal and become more physically active, you should consult your physician or other health-care professional before you begin. This is particularly true if you (or someone in your family) have a history of high blood pressure, diabetes, or heart disease.

By now you may be wondering, "What exactly is an affirmation?" Oxford Dictionary of English (2015) defines *affirmation* (a noun) as the action or process of affirming something. This definition is not as helpful without also understanding the definition of *affirm*: (a verb) to state as a fact; assert strongly and publicly. Oxford lists synonyms for *affirm*, including *declare, state, assert, proclaim, pronounce, attest,* and *swear*.

For the purposes of this book, the working definition of an affirmation is a little broader: the action of declaring something positive and helpful to yourself or to other people in a way that will bring about positive changes.

I have researched different formats of affirmations, and I settled on a hybrid version of a template by Hal Elrod (Elrod H., 2012). I've adapted this version for older adults. The question-and-answer format makes it easier to create new affirmations anytime you set a new goal or need some self-motivation to help you achieve a goal you are already working toward. I also find this affirmation outline flexible enough to apply to diverse needs and wants—whether they are physical, spiritual, or social. I've adapted Elrod's version for older adults with more emphasis on mindset, modifying step 4 with wearing a new "hat" (instead of taking on an entirely new identity, which is encouraged in other affirmation formats).

FIGURE 1 *AMAGING*™ AFFIRMATION OUTLINE

Step 1: What do you really want?
Step 2: What is your growth mindset to support this?
Step 3: Why do you want it?
Step 4: What new hat will you wear? Describe what type of person you are willing to become.
Step 5: What are you committed to doing? Be specific.
Step 6: Encourage yourself! Reinforce your affirmation with one or more inspirational quotes, proverbs, or words of scripture to build momentum and achieve your goal. Don't skimp on this step!

To illustrate how these steps come together to create an *Amaging*™ *Affirmation*, I've included examples throughout this book for you to use as is or to adapt to meet your needs. Use this format to write your own *Amaging*™ *Affirmation* and achieve your next goal. In appendix 1, I've included a fill-in-the-blank form to write your own *Amaging*™ *Affirmation* side by side with an action plan and a space for a mini vision board to help your mind's eye better picture yourself on the path to success. You can access a free fillable form for an *Amaging*™ *Affirmation* at www.amaging.info.

Step 1: Identify the problem you want to solve.

As with a lot of things, the first step is often the most challenging. We may know in our hearts something is not right, but it's not easy to pinpoint the exact problem worth solving. This may require reflection, research, asking friends, talking with a doctor or another expert, writing out a pros-and-cons chart, or all of the above. For example, before writing an affirmation on self-compassion, I had to identify that my self-talk warranted improvement. Before writing an affirmation on friendship, I had to identify that loneliness and isolation were issues for me. Before writing an affirmation called "Stuck on Savory," I had to identify that a diet without chocolate was actually a good thing.

Step 2: Pause and reflect on a growth mindset.

A growth mindset is a belief in the ability to grow, while a fixed mindset is a belief that things cannot or will not change. Ask yourself how you might reframe the situation that's running in your head in a more positive way. What new belief might help influence you to change your behavior to support this goal? For some people, a new mindset can come from a mentor or someone they look up to—and they adopt a similar mindset. A new mindset can also come about as you practice and develop new skills or as you take time to learn more about your goal and increase your understanding.

Here are a few questions to help you adopt a growth mindset:

- What belief (perhaps new to me) will move me in a positive direction toward solving my problem?
- What might I learn from this situation?
- What is the most important thing I may need to let go of in order to be successful here?
- What would help me push through in a positive direction?
- How would I describe my belief that this can be changed?

Step 3: Explore why you want this.

Ask yourself "why" a few times to get to the root cause for this change. Take time to reflect on what you realistically can control. You may even go so far as to consider how you wish to leave your legacy. Step 3 is discussed more in chapter 3.

Step 4: Select a new "hat" to wear.

When picking out this new hat, it is more important to consider the *process* of reaching your goal than the type of person you will be once you reach your goal. Give thought to the type of person who will be most successful with the *process*. As an example, if you have a goal to exercise more, you may come up with the idea to wear the hat of an athlete. However, take time to reflect on the *processes* followed by successful athletes. You may then decide you want to wear the hat of someone who can be consistent, someone who will come back and exercise the next day even if he missed the day before. If you have a goal to eat healthier, you may come up with the idea to wear the hat of a thin person. After reflecting on the *processes* followed by thinner people, you may want to wear the hat of a planner who writes a grocery list and shops in advance, so the refrigerator is well stocked with healthier "grab and go" foods.

When choosing which hat to wear, consider the *process* that's needed to reach your goal. What type of individual do you need to become in order to handle this new process?

Step 5: Create an action plan.

If you set a big, audacious goal, how will you get there? Affirm that you will take the many and consistent steps needed to be successful. If you are a linear thinker, this may be like connecting the dots from one to the next. Write out all the steps from beginning to end. If you are an organizer, here is your chance to open up a new spreadsheet and determine the line items needed to reach your best-possible bottom line. If your planning is normally more fragmented, you may want to grab a blank sheet of paper and draw a circle for each of your mini deadlines.

Then, within each circle, add a small cluster of activities you will do to meet each mini deadline before the big deadline.

There isn't a right or wrong way to action plan, as long as you make forward progress. Action planning is discussed more in chapter 6, "Setting *Amaging™* Goals as We Age."

Step 6: Encourage, give support, hope, and grow your confidence.

Sometimes to encourage is defined as "inspiring with courage." In her book, *Do it Scared*, Ruth Soukup outlines the different types of fear that often get in the way of progress. These range from the fear of making mistakes (the procrastinator), fear of authority (the rule stickler), fear of what others might think (the people pleaser), fear of rejection (the outcast), fear of adversity and of pain or struggle (the pessimist), fear of not being capable (self-doubter), to fear of taking responsibility (excuse maker).

You may find it helpful to reflect on your fears and to include encouraging thoughts, offsetting any fears as you develop step 6. Feel free to add another page or to use the back side of your *Amaging™ Affirmation* in your journal or notebook. Add as many pages as you need. For most of us, the need for encouragement is like a thirst that cannot be quenched. As Soukup writes:

> *As humans, we have an insatiable need for encouragement. It doesn't seem to matter how often we hear that we're smart or capable or beautiful or courageous or any other number of positive messages. We still need to hear it again and again.*

Keep hydrating your thirst for encouragement with your favorite quotes, inspiring stories, kind thoughts, Bible verses that speak to your situation, and other messages that resonate with you. Do not skimp on step 6!

It's important to practice affirmations daily. Twice a day is better than once a day. Three times a day is better than two. There is value in repetition. When you repeat a process, the neural connections in your brain grow stronger. Like learning any new skill, if you practice for even a few minutes each day, you will move closer toward your goal (Alidina, 2015). Zig Ziglar, a motivational speaker and author, is quoted as saying the following:

> People often say that motivation doesn't last. Well, neither does bathing—that's why we recommend it daily.

Think of affirmations as good hygiene for your goals. Use affirmations at least daily to clean out negative thoughts and to make progress toward your important goals (Alidina, 2015).

By now, I hope I've made a case for the value of affirmations. If not, here is a short summary of the benefits of affirmations as described in the book *Morning Sidekick Journal*. The authors suggest that affirmations will support goal setting in the following ways:

- tap into your creative side to help you think of creative options
- mentally sort out the steps needed
- envision yourself where you want to be
- motivate you to believe you have the ability and capability to do it (Atighehchi, Banayan, & Ahdoot, 2019)

Whether intentionally or unintentionally, successful people have used affirmations in all of these ways to achieve goals and be more successful. You can use them as well—at any age!

To stay on task while writing this book, I have needed some kindling, a match, and some fanning of the flames on occasion—similar to what I described regarding Lombardi Jr. in an earlier section. With my family, work, self-care, and other responsibilities, I couldn't write this book without finding the time to write it. This meant (gulp) becoming a morning person, not something that has come naturally for me in the past five-plus decades.

Here is an affirmation I wrote to help me achieve my goal of writing this manuscript (Figure 2). You'll notice I followed the *Amaging™ Affirmation* format.

FIGURE 2 *AMAGING*™ AFFIRMATION TO DO THE WRITE THING!

Step 1: What do you really want?

I want to complete a manuscript by [date] to submit to a publisher for editing and feedback. My ultimate goal is to write a nonfiction book to support wellness for older adults.

Step 2: What is your growth mindset to support this?

I believe I can learn and practice a daily writing habit.

Step 3: Why do you want it?

Too often elders, who may have lived a lifetime of ineffective or inconsistent habits, resign their thinking to accept the status quo with an attitude that it's too late to make changes. I want to expose a popular proverb as a myth: "You can't teach an old dog new tricks." In reality, older adults (including me) are learning new tricks all the time!

Step 4: What new hat will you wear? Describe what type of person you are willing to become.

Someone who consistently plans my day and carves out at least fifteen minutes per day, at the start or end of the day, to write.

Step 5: What are you committed to doing?

To meet my deadline, I am committed to write five to ten pages per week (or one or two pages per day). I will also read my "Rise and Shine" affirmation and this affirmation at least twice each day. I will replace my outdated laptop computer. I will study my vision board daily.

Step 6: Reinforce your affirmation with inspirational quotes, proverbs, or scripture:

We have different gifts, according to the grace given to each of us. If your gift is…serving, then serve; if it is teaching, then teach; if it is to encourage, <u>then give encouragement</u>; if it is giving, then give generously; if it is to lead, do it diligently; if it is to show mercy, do it cheerfully.

— Romans 12:7-9

Get it on the plate!

— Food Network
(Good intentions are not good enough. It's important to manage what little time I have in order to create something "edible" in a short amount of time.)

Ideas can come from anywhere at any time. The problem with making mental notes is that the ink fades rapidly.

—Rolf Smith
(Get my thoughts together, research done, and everything on paper.)

Can you see how this affirmation helped light a fire that helped me finish writing the manuscript? Of course, it was not enough to merely write the affirmation. I also had to discipline myself to read this affirmation often. Then, I had to apply what I read to my behaviors in the form of action planning, which is discussed more in chapter 6. This book will show you how affirmations can help you achieve your own important and *amaging*™ goals.

About Vision Boards

To reinforce your affirmations, you may wish to create a vision board accompanying your goals and affirmations. A vision board is simply a collection or collage of pictures representing your wishes or goals. A vision board can enhance your affirmations. It is another way to help get your mind in the right place for forming new daily habits and making gradual changes. Some people mix both words and pictures on their vision boards, but I prefer to use pictures alone to help reduce "message fatigue."

If this is something you wish to try, I recommend finding images that represent what you need to do to achieve your goal instead of images of the goal already accomplished. For example, if you have a goal to get up earlier each day, you may be tempted to use a photo of someone out of bed, fully dressed, and having coffee while the sun can be seen through a window, rising in the background. This would be a photo of your early-morning goal accomplished, which is less helpful than visualizing an image of someone pulling back the covers and stepping out of bed. Visualizing the processes needed for success will help you achieve your future vision.

For example, my vision board includes a collage with the following pictures I printed, cut, and pasted from the internet, including:

- Someone wearing pajamas with two feet on the ground, in the act of getting out of bed. This reinforces my "morning person" affirmation.
- Someone writing a list in a daily planner. I could have used an image of a well-used daily planner page, filled with scribbled notes and lists, but instead, I chose to show someone in the act of writing in the planner to support a consistent habit. Also, I didn't have any luck searching for this image online, so while holding my phone in my left hand, I took a photo of my right

hand in the act of writing in the planner. Excellent picture for my vision board!
- Fingers typing on a keyboard. I debated creating an image of this book with its cover jacket mocked up, as if it were a finished book. Instead, I decided to show the daily writing habit of my fingers typing away.
- A person standing in a kitchen with a cutting board and a pile of random vegetables, chopping a carrot. This demonstrates the habit of cleaning, cutting, and preparing vegetables, part of my goal to have healthy foods on hand.
- A woman lifting weights. This supports my goal to do more resistance training. I wanted to show the habit of lifting weights rather than a photo of a woman in a swimsuit with a toned and sculpted body.

You get the picture! If a vision board resonates with you, think of it as your own collection of images to support your current goals and affirmations. I created my vision board in a simple Word document and saved it on my desktop for easy access. I used the Crop function to do away with portions of any pictures that did not fit or might be distracting. For example, I usually crop out the faces of people in the pictures so it's easier for me to picture *myself* working toward the new habits.

My board has changed over time. For example, a few years ago, after a shoulder injury (an old injury, not the one I will talk about later in this book), I had an image on my vision board of a woman swimming the front crawl stroke in a lap pool. I had found I couldn't swim but a couple strokes without great pain, and my goal was to lap swim again. After several weeks of physical therapy and practice, I achieved this goal—hurray! Later, I deleted the photo and replaced it with a new image that represented a new goal. You don't need to do this electronically, either. If you have old magazines you are willing to cut apart, you can look for images and cut and glue them the old-fashioned way onto a piece of paper or cardboard.

Have some fun with your vision board and be creative.

In appendix 1 you'll find a fill-in-the-blank affirmation worksheet with space to insert an image. It's a one-page "trifecta" to help you set and achieve goals: 1) the affirmation, 2) goal with action steps, and 3) visual image—all on one page.

On the topic of self-limiting thoughts, Jack Canfield, co-author of the *Chicken Soup for the Soul* series, talks about the "Law of Attraction" and how powerful this law is. In one of his YouTube videos, he says, "If you focus on lack and negativity, then that is what will be attracted into your life." Negative messages can lead to depression, lower self-esteem, and lower self-confidence. Avoid affirmations such as, "Money is the root of all evil," and instead consider something like, "My life is abundant in every way."

Canfield suggests stating your desires in a positive way. Focus on the opposite of whatever you do *not* want. Rather than, "I don't want to get sick," give attention to good health. "I always enjoy being healthy, energetic, and strong," you might say. In general, affirmations are helpful when they focus on being well, positive, and optimistic. Avoid putting energy toward things you don't want in your life. (Canfield, YouTube, 2017). I followed this format when writing an affirmation to eat fewer sweets. The opposite of what I did not want (more sweets) is to eat more savory foods; hence, my affirmation, which I discuss more in chapter 11, is entitled, "Stuck on Savory."

In his book, *A Short Guide to a Long Life,* David B. Agus, MD, a pioneering cancer doctor and researcher, reveals innovative steps to help prolong the lives of his patients. Not surprisingly, Dr. Agus says he is a firm believer that hope and optimism are powerful forces. "How we think determines what we experience—good or bad. And nowhere is this truer than with our health," Agus says. He mentions his experience as a medical researcher and the "placebo effect"—when patients receive a placebo or harmless medicine, and it results in improved health outcomes. Agus attributes this placebo effect to a positive belief system. Similarly, in his experience, a negative belief system can lead to a downward spiral of poor health. "In general, people who approach their life optimistically do better in clinical trials…" Agus says. "If you believe that you can beat the odds and enjoy a long life, you just might."

To understand how affirmations can help change your life for the better, it may help to think about the interconnectedness involved with who we are, how we think, and what we do. Every day we are interconnected with others and events. Psychologist Kristin Neff, PhD, describes this in her book, *Self-Compassion: The Proven Power of Being Kind to Yourself* (Neff, 2015). More often it is outside circumstances, including your gene pool, that help form life patterns, according to Neff.

Think of yourself as the sum total of all of your prior circumstances, plus your economic and social background, culture, genetics, spirituality, and the people who you have been blessed to know. Neff suggests that too often we think we are self-contained units rather than an interconnected human being.

SCIENCE SUPPORTS AFFIRMATIONS

Social scientists have found that affirmations can be helpful in many ways. One study looked at how self-affirmations can assuage threats of stereotyping. By evaluating defensive reactions to situations that often threaten self-integrity, researchers found affirmations can ease these threats (Martens, Johns, Greenberg, & Schimel, 2006). During the research, participants self-evaluated their perceived strengths: relationships, creativity, humor, attractiveness, and other characteristics. In the study, participants self-identified their most important attribute and then wrote an essay describing why it was important. Researchers found this simple action of self-affirmation helped alleviate potentially negative stereotypes. This research was intended to better understand how members of stigmatized groups might begin to deal with stereotype threats.

Consider the benefits of affirmations to support older adults who face age bias, discussed later in this book. Stereotype threats impair self-integrity, and affirmations can repair them.

3

Why Do You Want It?

While all six steps to the *Amaging™ Affirmation* framework are important, it's essential that you put step 3 on paper, and that you write from your heart. Perhaps more than you first realize, the movement of thought from heart to paper will strengthen your affirmation. Consider a simplified root-cause analysis of your own goal. Ask yourself "why" five times. In my "Do the Write Thing" example above, I started with, "Because I want to finish something I started." Then I asked myself "why" again, and I said, "Because it's an important topic." Then I asked myself why it was an important topic, and I said to myself, "Older adults, myself included, sometimes think they are too old to do better." Then, after asking myself the fifth "why," I settled on "Too often elders, who may have lived a lifetime of ineffective or inconsistent habits, resign to accept the status quo with an attitude that it's too late to make changes. I want to expose a popular proverb as a myth: 'You can't teach an old dog new tricks.' In reality, older adults (including me) learn new tricks all the time."

Simon Sinek's bestseller, *Start with Why* and his popular Ted Talk address the importance of answering this "why" question. Sinek explores why some people and organizations are more innovative and more successful than others. He gives examples of great leaders in history who first started with "why" and then went on to set their goals and achieve their visions to bring about change. Sinek's *Start with Why* is intended to help people influence others. As you write your affirmations, use this same concept to influence yourself. Take time to pause and reflect on your personal why. Include a meaningful and thoughtful "why" in your own affirmations. You will inspire yourself to achieve your goals.

Uncover Your "Why," Change Your Legacy

Sometimes, inspiration can come from unexpected people. In 2018, on a recommendation from one of my wonderful siblings, I decided to volunteer for a prison ministry. For many weeks, I received a lesson packet in the mail with an inmate's Christianity lessons. As a volunteer tutor, I made any needed corrections and wrote comments on the lesson before sending the lesson packet back to the person in prison, along with a personal letter. When I first started as a volunteer, I wanted to help people. I have been a Christian as long as I can remember, raised in a conservative Christian home. I thought I might have something to offer people who didn't know Jesus, and I also thought it might help me to get a little "refresher course" to bolster my own faith each time I worked through the lessons—never a bad thing!

This did happen, and over time I also found that the contributions shared by people in prison have inspired me to rethink what matters most in my own life. While I have always tried to be a grateful person, I saw more clearly my many blessings, really big and very tiny ones, when I was a prison ministry volunteer. Today, I keep a brief log of the people I tutored, mostly to use as a prayer list, and I periodically review my list and pray for each one.

There's one name and one prayer request that stands out on this list. This prisoner's story touched my heart, and it reminded me that if we can change our thinking, we can change a lot, including our legacy. I'll call her "Sarah." In her lesson, Sarah was asked to reflect on the questions, "Who am I? Why am I here? Where am I going?" This was a highly reflective lesson! Sarah described her talent and ability to associate things that were happening with song lyrics. This became evident throughout her lesson, as she weaved in lyrics from some of her favorite songs within her essay questions. I was quite impressed, as it's hard for me to remember the exact words to songs, and I'm often guilty of making up lyrics as I sing along with the radio. Sarah knew many detailed lyrics, as well as the song titles and performers' full names.

Sarah said she needed to make some changes in her life, and she felt the combination of scripture, song lyrics, and affirmations would help her with her goals. In one of the action-planning sections in her lesson, Sarah said she had a goal to memorize key scriptures to recite whenever she has bad memories of past experiences with an abusive ex-husband. She struggled to keep these painful thoughts out of her head. Another action step Sarah shared was to, "Make affirmations from the truths in these lessons. Then recite these affirmations in the mirror every time I am in front of the mirror!" Sarah was tuned into the power of affirmations. Or, perhaps, she had good chaplains guiding her.

Because I was Sarah's tutor for this lesson, she shared how she had mapped out a new purpose for her life. Even while incarcerated and serving a life sentence, Sarah was a girl on a mission! She said she had always done what everyone else wanted her to do in life, but now she was chartering a new path to follow God's plan for her. When Sarah described why this mattered, she inspired me. Sarah was staying the course to leave a legacy. She said these lyrics embodied how she wanted people to remember her:

> *I want to leave a legacy,*
> *How will they remember me?*
> *Did I choose to love?*
> *Did I point to You enough?*
> *To make a mark on things*
> *I want to leave an offering*
> *A child of mercy and grace*
> *Who blessed Your name unapologetically*
> *And leave that kind of legacy.* (Howard, 2002)

Of course, Sarah may have been exaggerating, but her words seemed to come from her heart. Sarah has a big, audacious goal to leave a legacy. I continue to keep her on my prayer list. I pray that she will find a way to forgive her ex-husband, that she will remain focused on her goals, and that her gift to remember song lyrics along with daily affirmations will help Sarah to leave a legacy of someone whose love for Jesus turned an angry heart into a loving one—and restored her soul.

What Do You Have Control Over?

In his book, *The Virtues of Aging*, former President Jimmy Carter described some of the challenges he faced during the immediate months after leaving the White House. Not only had he lost his job in a very public way, but he and his wife, Rosalyn, had also suffered great agriculture losses and considered selling the family farm. In their middle fifties, they felt that their lives had spun out of control.

> We did not yet understand there were potential advantages ahead of us, if we could only put to use the good advice we received, along with our personal assets, the support of friends and family, and some courage and planning (Carter, 1998).

The Carters took control of the situations that they *could* control and reinvented themselves. Both had offers to become university professors, to author books, to establish The Carter Center, and to take on other new challenges. Along the way, they came to realize their primary purpose wasn't just living as long as possible, but also to enjoy living.

Here is another example of focusing on what you can control: At age 51 and after learning her neighbor was killed and a victim of domestic violence, Sue Rock in Brooklyn, New York, was inspired to action. Rock learned her neighbor had filed a protection order with law enforcement, but later died a violent death at the hands of her spouse. Sue and her husband were shocked and subsequently gave much thought to how they could combine their talents to help struggling victims of domestic violence. Both had experience in the clothing industry, and they realized victims of violence often flee with just the clothes on their backs. This story is described by Marlo Thomas in her book, *It Ain't Over… Till It's Over*. Rock and her husband formed a charity, Sue Rock Originals Everyone, Inc., and the charity encouraged communities to support violence victims with clothing—a comforting and meaningful gift (Thomas, 2014).

Rock's charity has been featured on *Sewing with Nancy*, a popular Wisconsin Public Television program for needle arts. According to SueRock.com, the charity has donated more than 450 quilts to domestic violence survivors in New York City; it has given fabric and underwear to young girls in twelve developing countries; and the charity has made other sewing-related contributions, including teaching victims how to sew. While the Rocks could not put an end to domestic violence, they gave attention to what they knew and felt they could control—comfortable clothing for women who really need it. Then, one stitch at a time, they began to help others.

What do you Enjoy Doing?

Have you ever been working on a project and lost sense of time, only to look at your watch and realize it was much later than you expected? Have you ever offered to do something from which others emphatically turned away, but you didn't mind because you rather enjoyed it? On the flip side, have you ever found that a chunk of free time was less enjoyable than you thought it would be, because it took a fair amount of energy to make it meaningful? Deeply engaging in an activity that you enjoy doing is a special thing.

I enjoy cooking. If I invite people over for a meal, the "work" involved usually means cleaning and making my house somewhat presentable for guests. Kitchen tasks like peeling, cutting, measuring, stirring, cooking, and baking are fun for me. I even enjoy shopping for groceries. When

I plan a menu, stir a stir-fry, or bake a pan of dinner rolls, I lose sense of time. The work is not too easy that I get bored nor too difficult that I start to dislike it. While cooking, I'm in what psychologist Mihaly Csikszentmihalyi describes as a state of "flow." Flow occurs when the challenge of the activity matches your skill, and your mind is focused and feels some sense of serenity, creativity, timelessness—and enjoyment (Csikszentmihalyi, 2008).

As an older adult, when you reflect on new habits, lifestyle changes, and goals you want to achieve, take some time to consider what stretches you. Csikszentmihalyi says, "Contrary to what we usually believe, moments like these (optimal experiences), the best moments in our lives, are not the passive, receptive, relaxing times—although such experiences can be enjoyable… The best moments usually occur when a person's body or mind is stretched to its limits in a voluntary effort to accomplish something difficult and worthwhile."

A key word here is *voluntary*. You have the control, and you select what brings you joy. For many people, this joy comes from making things happen. Take time to reflect on what you enjoy. What is a mindful challenge for you, and one you also enjoy doing? For some this may be time spent walking on a nature trail, putting puzzles together, practicing piano, doing yoga, tinkering with woodworking, quilting, or any time spent visiting with family. These are just a few examples. Everyone is different. *What brings you joy?*

As you create your *Amaging™ Affirmations*, it is perfectly okay to answer the question, "Why do I want it?" with a response like, "Because it's fun for me!" When you are in a state of flow with a purpose, and you make progress, this helps the task feel more fun and easier. Look for a balance between easy and difficult to help you get more absorbed in your goals and feel a sense of timelessness and enjoyment.

On this topic of "why," if you visit your health-care provider and learn you have bad test results, such as high blood pressure, high cholesterol, or high blood sugar levels, your personal "why" may be to lower the numbers and improve your health. Your health-care team may give you the "why," along with recommended goals to guide your action planning. In chapter 11, I talk about better food habits to pursue while aging, and I share my personal "why" I set healthy food habits when my labs came back after an annual wellness exam.

Is your Purpose Hiding? Go Find It!

At young ages, some people have found ways to lead purpose-filled lives and follow a course to achieve this purpose pretty consistently. Consider the example of an elementary school teacher who very early in life decided she wanted to teach and mentor young children. This teacher's career and life were devoted to the care and learning of elementary school children.

Later, in retirement years, the teacher cherished time spent mentoring and caring for grandchildren, or perhaps young children in her neighborhood. This teacher's purpose to teach and mentor youth never wavered. For others, our purpose may have changed or pivoted when life brought on new challenges or opportunities. In chapter 9, which focuses on friendship, I tell a story about Jeff Krause, a high school choir director. I have no doubt he knew at a young age that his life's purpose would relate to music, teaching, and possibly also to building friendships.

In life, we may have had high points and low points that combined to shape who we are. The National Council on Aging promotes a program entitled, "Aging Mastery," which includes six dimensions of aging well, including identifying "legacy and purpose" to make the most out of the gift of time on this earth. The Aging Mastery program recommends that participants find a purpose larger than themselves, and it advocates that it is this type of purpose that helps people thrive in their later years. Here are the three main steps recommended by Aging Mastery® to help older adults reflect upon, and then take action on, life's purpose (Firman, 2018):

1. Reflect on your responsibilities and your life's purpose
2. Create the pathway for your life's purpose to flourish
3. Build your legacy by serving others, teaching, and storytelling

These three steps remind me of Neil Armstrong's famous quote when he first walked on the moon, "One small step for a man, one giant leap for mankind." The authors of Aging Mastery® have brilliantly broken purpose-finding into three steps. Yet, these are not easy steps to tackle; they are incredibly big steps, and, when combined, can be giant leaps.

If reflecting on and then building your purpose seems pretty formidable, you may want to think in smaller terms, like a mission. A mission does not need to bring about world peace nor impact entire communities—it just needs to be something that is meaningful to you and touches your heart. In his book, *The Miracle Equation,* Hal Elrod describes a formula anyone can use to help them do miraculous things with their lives. While it isn't a key element in the formula, Elrod says articulating your mission is a good way to help maintain your enthusiasm and faith that you can accomplish what you want to accomplish. "The missing link between wanting something and attaining it is often leverage, and your deeply meaningful *why* will give you that leverage," Elrod says. He suggests we take time to articulate our *why:*

- What are the most significant benefits?
- Who will you become if you attain it?

For example, this could be better relationships, a healthier physical body, financial rewards, or other benefits.

This book focuses on the *amaging*™ purposes and possibilities within all of us, the use of affirmations to support our goals while growing older, and the need for affirmations to help offset our anti-aging culture. This anti-aging culture is discussed more in the next chapter on age bias.

4

Become More Aware of Age Bias

"A good start to adding more good years to your life would be to get rid of the anti-aging quackery."
—Tom Perls, New England Centenarian Study

Aging is a relatively new experience in the history of people. In 1940, when Social Security was implemented in the United States, the average life expectancy was just 58. Let that sink in a little bit. Only those who lived to age 65 would be able to claim the benefits of Social Security. Fast-forward approximately eight decades, and the world as we know it is very different. The miracles of public utilities, modern agriculture, medical research, and technology have contributed to the luxuries of better hygiene, well-stocked grocery stores, and highly specialized medical technology and experts. While our great-great-great grandparents likely died more suddenly due to an infectious disease or a serious injury, today's generations are living considerably longer.

Today, what's eventually killing us is not usually sudden but rather a chronic or ongoing health problem, or multiple chronic problems spread out over many years. For some of us, ongoing health conditions zap our physical capabilities and chip away at our growth mindset and our positive attitudes toward aging.

This chipping-away business is often unnoticed and not discussed. We likely do not talk about growing older outside of our birthdays or our annual physical exams. Like politics, religion, sex, personal finances, illegal drugs, alcoholism, adultery, and other taboo subjects, our advancing age is not usually part of polite conversation. Similarly, age bias has been a taboo topic. Age bias, also called ageism, is defined as a systematic stereotyping of and discrimination against people on the basis of their age (North, 2015). A common example of age bias is the general assumption that all older adults become mentally and physically incapacitated.

Actually, the overwhelming majority of older adults are not incapacitated. Unlike other prejudices, age bias is more socially acceptable, and, if we live long enough, age bias will eventually target every one of us.

Virtually everyone strives to live a long time, while simultaneously moving toward joining a (mostly) undesirable social group.
—Michael S. North, an expert on age bias *(North, 2015)*.

A landmark study on aging perceptions conducted and reported by the Frameworks Institute in Washington, DC, was organized by eight champions for older adults in the United States:

- American Federation for Aging Research
- American Geriatrics Society
- American Society on Aging, Grantmakers in Aging
- Gerontological Society of America
- National Council on Aging
- National Hispanic Council on Aging
- American Association of Retired Persons

Funding for the study came from the collaborative's supporters, including the Retirement Research Foundation, the John A. Hartford Foundation, and others. The study identified three broad categories of misperceptions regarding older adult:

1. Misperception: Aging equals inevitable decline.
2. Misperception: Older adults are seen as "others," often compartmentalized outside the rest of society.
3. Misperception: Culpability, elders are accountable for their circumstances. The well-being of older adults is exclusively the result of individual lifestyle choices and financial planning.

In the 2015 report titled, "Gauging Aging," the Frameworks Institute found prevalent thinking was very different from what aging experts had to say:

> *The experts…emphasized that aging is not synonymous with disease or disability. With the right contextual and social supports, older adults remain healthy and maintain high levels of independence and function.*

When we think decline is inevitable and a "normal part of aging," we may develop a mindset based on the notion that nothing can be done, or a "Why bother?" attitude. The experts interviewed by Frameworks also said (and I hope those of you reading this book agree) that older adults are an integral part of society with enormous economic and social impact that often goes under-recognized. Finally, in the Frameworks report, experts identified public policy, employment opportunities, and social determinants as working together to support a good quality of life for elders.

If you have read this book from the beginning, you have noticed that I examine the power of the individual's mindset, positive thinking and words, affirmations, and individual action planning. At the same time, I do want to recognize the value of societal support for the aging sector. Individualism—choice, planning ahead, self-control, individual responsibility—are *not* the sole factors. Interventions to support older adults are needed. Examples of these interventions include public policy, employment policies, and practices to help older adults. If this is a topic in which you are interested, I encourage you to read the full report, *Gauging Aging: Mapping the Gaps between Expert and Public Understandings of Aging in America* (Lindland E., 2016).

We'll talk more about the importance of having a positive attitude later in this chapter. First, I want to describe what a negative attitude toward aging looks like. Unfortunately, many people dread aging. I remember my mother saying that she was still twenty-nine well into her fourth and fifth decades, and (of course) I did the same when I got older—until I became a student of age bias. It's part of our culture to dislike old age, even though aging is a privilege. I lost a brother who was just nineteen years old, so I very much understand what is meant by the saying, "Growing old is a privilege denied to many."

There are many people who have lost loved ones far too young due to automobile crashes, cancer, heart disease, suicide, and other life-ending perils that have mercilessly denied individuals the privilege of aging. Yet, our culture dreads and doesn't cherish old age. We idealize the concept of being "forever young," while our entire society pretty much denies death, dying, and getting older.

When Jimmy Carter wrote *The Virtues of Aging*, which I mentioned earlier, he said some people he talked with about the manuscript would say things like, "Virtues? What could possibly be good about growing old?" While it was nearly twenty years ago that Carter wrote his book, I doubt public perception has changed much for the better. Today, an anti-aging bias continues. Sadly, older adults frequently hold this bias toward themselves—and toward other elders who are their friends, loved ones, and people they generally care about. It is so much a part of our culture that we often may not notice it. It's an unconscious bias.

Age bias can also be a tendency to regard older persons as debilitated, unworthy of attention, or unsuitable for employment (Dictionary.com, 2019). I have also heard ageism defined as a prejudice against our future self. Ouch! It is an "-ism" by which everyone who lives long enough will be affected, and it's likely one of the few "-isms" that are still socially acceptable. Consider the popular birthday cards that have a picture of a well-worn older adult on the cover and then a derogatory comment about aging on the inside, along with a happy birthday message! Many of us have sent or received one of these cards, and we see similar content floating in and out of our social media feeds as a matter of routine. Now, substitute the aging imagery with imagery for a person of color, a person of a certain religion, or a homosexual. Would greeting cards or social media posts that poke fun at these groups of people be socially acceptable? Considered funny? Marketable?

So, why do we laugh at jokes and cartoons that poke fun at elders?

You may think that I am being extreme or that I've lost my sense of humor. I hope it's evident by now that I have a sense of humor. Yet, since I learned more about the prevalence of age bias and why it matters so much, especially for our health, I have moved old-age jokes and greeting cards out of the funny column. I think it's sad when a society finds humor in belittling our elders. Instead, we should be lifting them up, celebrating them, learning from them, and appreciating them.

UNCONSCIOUS BIAS AGAINST AGING

As the term implies, *unconscious* is unaware and usually unintentional. It can be automatic when our minds are not fully present. Often, we think of biases relating to ethnicity and race; however, unconscious biases also relate to gender, religion, sexual orientation, weight, and many other characteristics including age. A bias is a prejudice, either in favor of or against something. I like to think I am *consciously* bias toward older adults, looking for their best and *amaging*™ attributes! You may not realize this, but everyone holds unconscious beliefs about various groups, and these biases stem from our established tendencies to categorize things.

This book includes examples of affirmations for older adults to help offset our anti-aging culture. Because age bias is often unconscious and not intentional, it may be hard to pinpoint in your community or in the news and social media sources you access. Here are some ways unconscious age bias is prevalent:

- Age prejudice in advertising that portrays older adults as frail, slow, with poor cognition, etc.
- Marketing strategies that target those age 65 and older yet include images of people who are much younger. Interestingly, it is older adults who have more disposable income to purchase goods than their younger counterparts.
- Management practices that encourage retirement or make promotion decisions based on age.
- Assumptions that all older adults are disabled. While disability is common among older adults, nearly two-thirds of adults over age 65 report no disabilities.
- Assumptions that growing old should be dreaded or feared.

In my career, the marketing strategy of showing images of younger adults when targeting an older demographic has been particularly frustrating. I realize this is because marketers want to include images consumers aspire toward. Yet, are aspirations not shaped by advertising?

Want to Live Longer? Change your Attitude about Aging

A negative attitude about growing older can have a negative impact on health. Much research has been done in this field by Dr. Becca Levy, Yale University, who has published a number of studies on this topic. Using an "attitudes toward own aging" assessment scale, Levy found those with low expectations for aging were less likely to participate in prevention activities like a regular physical exam, good nutrition, wearing a seatbelt, exercising, and limiting alcohol or tobacco (Ouchida, 2015).

Those who had positive perceptions about aging were more likely to engage in preventive health behaviors, had better functional health, and were 44 percent more likely to fully recover from a severe disability when compared with those who had negative age stereotypes. Levy's findings also showed those who held more optimistic views of aging lived 7.5 years longer than those with less positive perceptions (Ouchida, 2015).

The cardiologists who treat heart conditions, the orthopedic specialists who repair bones and joints, the oncologists who care for older adult cancer patients, and all the talented health-care providers who specialize in their respective body parts and conditions, may flinch at the fact that this research found something as simplistic as a positive attitude adds more years to life than some of the complex and costly interventions they prescribe. Yet, it is hard to dispute that Levy's 7.5 years is based on high-level evidence from randomized and controlled trials.

Do you want to enhance your wellness regimen? Consider the ways you might give more attention to a positive attitude toward aging. After some time for reflection, perhaps write out some helpful steps. In appendix 1, I've included a fill-in-the-blank form to write your own *Amaging™ Affirmation*, and in Figure 3, below, I share an example.

Growing Older and Becoming More Different

The older we get, the more different from other people we become. I'll just repeat that for emphasis: The older we get, the more different from other people we become. What are some of the reasons society collectively stereotypes an extremely diverse sector? Ashton Applewhite is an ageism expert and author who is actively tackling the subject of unintentional age bias. Applewhite has authored, *This Chair Rocks*, a book that shows how ageism twists our view of old age. Her writings encourage readers to challenge age-biased prejudices both in society and in ourselves.

Fortunately, Applewhite offers remedies for age bias. She suggests three antidotes we can use to be more positive about aging:

- **Awareness**. Learn more about aging and unconscious age bias. From your studies, you may find some of the personal problems you face are common societal problems. An example of this might be an inability to find a job after age 60, being disrespected in a grocery store checkout line while carefully (albeit slowly) using your bank card, or generally feeling patronized.
- **Integration**. Connect with people of all ages, young and old. Learn from each other. If we spend the majority of our time with people who are just like us, we miss opportunities to find shared connections.
- **Activism**. Challenge age bias when you see it. Support every stage of life's journey. Whether it is a derogatory cartoon as you scroll through social media, a new policy where you work that makes assumptions about older adults, or a marketing campaign that stereotypes elders, when you see it, name it as age bias.

I would add curiosity and affirmations to this antidote list:

- **Curiosity**. Ask questions and wonder if age bias might be present. Ask questions of others and especially of yourself. Why is this the status quo? Could we do better for older adults? Could *I* do better if *I* reframe *my* point of view? If I were more positive? Are these assumptions based on fact or appropriate past experiences? Or are they based on emotion? Perhaps they are based on my own fear of growing older? Let curiosity help point you toward a positive change.
- *Amaging*™ *Affirmations.* Use the *Amaging*™ *Affirmations* described in this book. This book focuses on the *amaging*™

possibilities within all of us, the use of affirmations to support our goals while growing older, and the need for affirmations to help offset our anti-aging culture.

Here's an *Amaging™ Affirmation* to help you be more positive about aging, to be more aware of age bias, to challenge age bias, and to use curiosity to help you achieve your goals as you grow older. Feel free to adapt this and make it your own *Amaging™ Affirmation*.

Figure 3 *Amaging™ Affirmation*: Be More Positive about Growing Older

Step 1: What do you really want?

I want to be more positive about growing older.

Step 2: What is your growth mindset to support this?

I can learn, grow, and change my own attitude about aging, and this can help me not only live longer but also to more fully enjoy this part of life's journey.

Step 3: Why do you want it?

My opportunities have not vanished; I want to keep pursuing them. I want to rekindle an "I think I can" spirit and use it to make the most of each day.

Step 4: What new hat will you wear? Describe what type of person you are willing to become.

I will become a learner and learn about age bias and the detriment of negative attitudes about growing older. I will become a more curious friend, looking for opportunities to make connections with people of all ages. I will become a person with more courage to speak up and call out age bias when it is suspected or likely. I will speak up with kindness, humility, and decency.

Step 5: What are you committed to doing? Be specific.

I will finish reading this book to understand how to be more *amaging*™—then return to this book later as needed for a refresher. I will read this affirmation routinely, and I will attend programs and events to socialize with people of all ages. Lastly, I will take time to reflect on past ideas and potential goals I may have set aside due to my own ageist thoughts and attitudes. I will take time to consider whether there are projects, activities, groups, or other things I might now revisit with an "I think I can" attitude. I will set *amaging*™ goals.

Step 6: How will you encourage yourself?

Reinforce your affirmation with one or more inspirational quotes, proverbs, or scripture to build momentum and achieve your goal. Don't skimp on this step!

> *Finally, brothers and sisters, whatever is true, whatever is noble, whatever is right, whatever is pure, whatever is lovely, whatever is admirable—if anything is excellent or praiseworthy—think about such things.*
>
> —Philippians 4:8

> *Our (research) findings make a strong case for efforts aimed at reducing the epidemic of ageism, which produces not only a financial cost for society but also a human cost for the well-being of older persons.*
>
> —Becca Levy, PhD, Yale University

> *Optimism is the faith that leads to achievement. Nothing can be done without hope and confidence.*
>
> —Helen Keller

"In general, people who approach their life optimistically do better in clinical trials. ... If you believe that you can beat the odds and enjoy a long life, you just might,"

—David Agus, MD

"I want to avoid slotting people into a category based on age and help people overcome a feeling of being stuck due to age."

—Margie Hackbarth, Amaging™ Growing Old On Purpose

5

More Than Fluff

The topic of affirmations may sound like fluff or trivial. If you're a fan of TV's *Saturday Night Live* (SNL), you may think affirmations are at best comical and at worst a waste of time! The popular SNL skits with Al Franken portrayed a fictional self-help evangelist named Stuart Smalley. You may remember one of Smalley's frequent quotes, "I'm good enough. I'm smart enough, and doggone it, people like me!" Some of Smalley's other often-used quotes include:

- "That's just stinkin' thinkin'!"
- "You're should-ing all over yourself."
- "You need a checkup from the neck up." (Saturday Night Live, n.d.)

"These are pretty cheesy!" as my youngest daughter would say! Those who thought this is what they were getting into when they started reading this book have perhaps stopped reading. But you're still here! The sample affirmations in this book are different. Admittedly they are focused on self-help, but that is probably the only similarity to Smalley's quotes or skits. The affirmations I've written in this book follow a series of questions and emphasize *why* you believe it's important to move yourself to action and what new hat you are willing to wear. What new type of person are you willing to become in order to accomplish what you want to accomplish?

Affirmations to support personal goals are based on evidence. A study done at Brock University in Ontario, Canada, and published by the American College of Sports Medicine describes the effectiveness of self-talk on athletes' heat tolerance while performing in the heat. Researchers studied eighteen cyclists and measured their executive function, reaction times, and memory. They found motivational self-talk significantly improved both speed and accuracy for executive functions. Executive functions are a set of cognitive processes needed to control behaviors and accomplish goals (Wallace, et al., 2017).

Evidence shows that self-affirmation influences health-promoting behaviors in a good way. *Health Psychology* published a study about this (Epton, 2008). In this all-female study, women used self-affirmations relating to acts of kindness prior to messages relating to the health benefits of fruits and vegetables. Researchers measured the test subjects' intentions to eat healthier as well as their fruit and vegetable consumption. On average, the self-affirmed participants ate more portions of fruit and vegetables when compared with the control group.

In another report, researchers at the University of Michigan studied the brain's response to health messages and any subsequent behavior changes among sedentary adults (Falk, 2015). For the purposes of this study, sedentary was defined as less than 195 minutes per week of walking, moderate, and vigorous physical activity. During one phase of the study, participants received one health message per day and then one "value affirmation" per day. The team found, on average, that patients showed a significant decline in sedentary behavior during the month after affirmations were utilized. Those exposed to the affirmations also exercised more.

A study published in 2009 in *Health Psychology* explored how self-affirmations affect responses to stressors (Sherman, 2009). The interventions helped vulnerable individuals draw on self-resources to improve their responses to natural stressors. This study was based on a theory that people can be affirmed by engaging in activities that remind them of who they are. In one part of the study, students affirmed their important values, and doing so helped buffer them during a stressful exam period.

Self-affirmation and the role of positive feelings were also described in *Psychological Science* in 2008. Researchers found affirmations with values, things people care about (beyond themselves) and that are more than temporary feelings, helped people rise above difficult situations. The studies suggest that reminding people what they love or care about may enable them to foster new learning under difficult circumstances (Crocker, 2008).

A more detailed review of self-affirmation can be found in a 2014 article found in the *Annual Review of Psychology*, (Cohen & Sherman, 2014). In this article, self-affirmations are described simply as an act that demonstrates one's adequacy. Self-affirmations were found helpful for both big and small accomplishments. Some of the examples given include a stressed employee who cares for his children and who may self-affirm by reflecting on the personal importance of his family. An ill resident in a nursing home may self-affirm by taking control over daily visitations (by deciding who is allowed to visit the resident). In one example, a small affirmation was found to have a big impact when a lonely patient received a kind note from a doctor and realized that other people care about her.

During times of high stress or threats to the self, well-timed self-affirmations can "help people navigate difficulties and set them on a better path." Interestingly, these well-timed self-affirmations are also impactful as they increase a person's self-confidence in their abilities to overcome future difficulties. This can then "bolster coping and resilience for the next adversity, in a self-reinforcing narrative." (Cohen & Sherman, 2014).

When we bring forward the power of affirming words at key moments, we can not only overcome the immediate obstacle, but also better prepare for future obstacles.

WHIMSICAL WORDS WITH A SERIOUS MESSAGE

Even whimsical words can be powerful. Word choices may mean very little to others, but a lot to you. Words may sound silly but have a serious meaning. For example, the phrase "The chicken runs at midnight" was coined by Amy Donnelly, the late daughter of Rich Donnelly, a professional baseball coach. In his Pittsburgh Pirates position as a third-base coach, Donnelly would crouch down and squat, cupping his hands over his mouth to yell messages to second-base runners. For those watching, Donnelly's communication couldn't be interpreted. Only the players knew the coach's message. The family sometimes joked about what he actually said. Amy asked him if he was just saying something like, "The chicken runs at midnight." At the time she was a teenager and enjoyed repeating this silly mantra. Soon others in the family joined in. It became the family's inside joke (Friend, 2018).

Unfortunately, Amy died in 1993 of cancer at the age of 18. Four years later, Rich took a new job with the Florida Marlins, which had a second baseman named Craig Counsell (now the manager of the Milwaukee Brewers). Because Craig was tall and skinny with an unusual high-armed batting stance, he earned a nickname of "Chicken Man."

Donnelly took his two sons to work with him as batboys when feasible, and they were present when the team continued into the playoffs that season. During the seventh game of the last playoff series, the team played late into the night in extra innings. It was an important game, as the winner would advance to the World Series, and the loser would be done for the season.

In the bottom of the eleventh inning, Craig Counsell was batted in and crossed home plate to win the game. As the team celebrated on the field, one of Rich's sons (a batboy) looked up at the clock and noticed it was midnight. He ran to his father to let him know, "Dad, the chicken ran at midnight!" (Friend, 2018).

Rich has since told this story and said if he had quit coaching after his daughter's death, he never would have made it to the World Series or experienced the way his daughter's presence was felt when the "Chicken," Craig Counsell, ran home to win the game at midnight. While he would have much preferred his daughter to be there in person to celebrate the win, he felt she was there in spirit with him, with his family, and with the team that night.

I like this story, and not just because Craig Counsell was my favorite utility player and a hometown athlete who returned to coach the Milwaukee Brewers. I can appreciate how this story demonstrates that words, even silly ones, can become something meaningful. While Amy coined the phrase as a way of making people laugh, her phrase meant different things to different people—perhaps the importance of family and the value of small joys.

Your personal affirmations do not need to be serious as long as they have a deeper meaning to you.

THE POWER OF WORDS IN A BAD WAY

Just as positive words can impact our lives and others favorably, negative words can be detrimental. Consider the unwelcomed visit to a family doctor after test results are found to be abnormal. If you have been fortunate to never get a bad diagnosis, you can only imagine how words like *cancer, dementia, surgery, organ failure, amputation,* or *terminal* might have the power to turn relatively calm emotions into extreme ones almost immediately. Emotions like sadness, shock, confusion, or even rage might suddenly take over when the upsetting words are heard. Words can influence more than emotions. In this example of a bad diagnosis, just hearing the life-changing words might cause a body to respond *physically*, involuntarily moving someone to actions like crying, shaking, being unable to speak, or even fainting.

Less obvious may be the negativity that comes from verbal abuse, which is a type of violence. While not physical, this type of abuse can be painful and cause injury. A study of more than 93,600 women by the Women's Health Initiative (WHI) Observational Study found higher incidents of depression among those who experienced the mental anguish of yelling, screaming, threatening, humiliating, and other verbal abuses. The women studied were ages 50 to 79. Women who had experiences of emotional abuse were found to have lower scores on physical function and general health. The researchers recommended early detection and taking steps to alleviate abusive situations, which can have important benefits for overall quality of life. This recommendation was based on a three-year study with a large number of older adult women (Mouton, Rodabough, Rovi, Brzyski, & Katerndahl, 2010).

Verbal abuse is an extreme example of the negative impact of negative words. Sometimes the negativity in our language is less extreme, yet still detrimental. Here are a few examples of negativity that might slip into our language and damage relationships:

> Using **extreme verbs,** like "hate." if you don't like Brussel sprouts, consider saying, "I haven't learned to like Brussel sprouts," instead of "I hate Brussel sprouts." Growing up, my parents made a big deal out of this at the dinner table. We were not allowed to use the word *hate*, and we would be stopped midsentence to replace *hate* with "I haven't learned to like Brussels sprouts." This was true regardless of what we wanted to describe—a food, an activity, a thing, a person, or anything. *Hate* is extreme, and if you find yourself using this word, consider it a red flag to stop yourself, reflect, and ask whether you might be acting judgmentally. On this topic, consider the synonyms for

hate that may sound less severe or more sophisticated, such as *detest, abhor, despise,* etc. These are red flags as well.

Using **extreme words that indicate frequency**, like *always* or *never*. Sometimes we are quick to say things *always* go a certain way or *never* go the way we want. We may perceive someone *always* does a certain thing or *never* helps in a certain way. This is likely not true! When we use extreme words, we condition our minds to look past the exceptions, which may be very exceptional, very favorable, and may take place far more frequently than our mind allows us to observe.

Negative descriptions of **perceived character weaknesses**. Similar to *always* and *never*, when we label a person as a *jerk, evil, arrogant,* or *annoying,* etc., our minds become conditioned to the label, and we look past the good in others. While it may be necessary to describe a person's behaviors, it's best to avoid labeling the person in a bad way. A recent action may have been *idiotic*, but the person who did this action is not an *idiot*. A child may do a *naughty* act, but the child doesn't deserve the label *naughty*. There is a difference! Also, ask yourself if it's truly necessary to describe a person's negative traits. Remember my friend Ginny's motto: If you can't find something nice to say about someone, don't say it at all.

Negative labels for ourselves. Just as we don't want to give someone else a negative label, we don't want to give ourselves one. An unintentional consequence could likely occur, and you might live out the label you've given yourself. Talk to yourself just as kindly and respectfully as you would talk to your neighbor.

If you have struggled with extreme words in your vocabulary, you may want to write an affirmation to help avoid it. Write an action plan to improve how you talk about others or how you talk about yourself this week. Take small and consistent steps to change your words for the better. Start today! In chapter 2, I shared an outline to help you create your own *Amaging™ Affirmation* to support your personal goals. Appendix 1 includes a template for an easy-to-follow action plan. You can access a free fillable form for an *Amaging™ Affirmation* at www.amaging.info.

6

Setting Amazing™ Goals as We Age

"Life begins at the end of your comfort zone."
—Neale Donald Walsch

Sometimes the unthinkable happens, and we are faced with a crisis or disaster so bad that it's hard to imagine how to move forward. This was the case for Scott Rigsby, a young athlete who was seriously injured in a vehicle accident, leaving him with one leg amputated and the other badly injured. The remaining leg caused ongoing pain. He tells his life story in the book, *UnThinkable*. Shortly after his accident, Rigsby recalled, "Nothing about my life was going to be the way I had planned it." He had learned to adjust to his new physical limitations. Rigsby suffered a traumatic brain injury that required multiple surgeries and caused panic attacks, constant pain, depression, and later a sleeping disorder. Rigsby found himself on a misguided path for more than a decade before reluctantly agreeing to have his second leg amputated as a solution for diminishing the pain.

After his horrific accident and throughout his young adult life, Rigsby struggled in the workforce and moved from job to job with stints for medical leaves in between. Then, something happened at age 37, almost nineteen years after Rigsby's accident. He had accepted that his high school best athletic days were long behind him. He knew he could not go back in time. He had never been an endurance athlete, but he had a desire to train and compete in an Ironman Triathlon. He was a Christian who believed God's timing was perfect, and while he questioned his own desires, he trusted in God's timing.

Rigsby also had an affirmation: "Do what you can, do the best you can, and don't ever quit," (Rigsby, 2009). He started running and walking with the help of prosthetic limbs and in his church parking lot where he felt less visible to passersby. Each day he tried to run a little more than the day before. After he was comfortable running, he began to learn how to ride a bike and swim. He'd learned how to do both as a child, but now he had to learn how to swim and bike with prosthetics. Rigsby said showing up and putting in the hours was essential to train well. He also learned to value mental training and commitment. He found ways to overcome excuses and even overcome legitimate reasons to skip training.

Rigsby endured many challenges, including his prosthetics breaking down, money problems, and open wounds where his prosthetics were attached. Yet, he forged ahead and continued to train, despite misfortune and ailments. In 2007, after two years of training, Rigsby did the unthinkable: he crossed the finish line and became the first double amputee to complete the world-famous Hawaiian Ironman Triathlon. I recommend this book to anyone looking for motivation to set and achieve a goal.

According to his LinkedIn profile, Rigsby is the founder of the Scott Rigsby Foundation, a Georgia-based nonprofit organization created to inspire and enable physically challenged individuals and athletes. He's described as a gifted counselor to people who have experienced pain and loss. Rigsby identified a set of five steps (Rigsby, 2009) to achieve his goal of participating in the Ironman competition, and he encourages others to set goals and follow these steps.

I advocate Rigsby's five steps to achieving a goal. They are life lessons for older adults who may wrongly think their best days are behind them.

- Expect and overcome obstacles.
- Build a good support team.
- Choose faith over fear.
- Cross your finish line. Your personal finish line may be unthinkable, initially. Try anyway!
- Have a dream. What is big in your heart and driving you? Does it seem unattainable right now? Follow it anyway. (Rigsby, 2009).

Rigsby's fifth step may be the most powerful for older adults. It's okay to have dreams later in life—at any age. It's similar to Step 5 in the framework for *Amaging™ Affirmations*: What are you committed to doing? Be specific.

I sometimes co-lead a "Living Well with Chronic Conditions" workshop. In it, participants set goals at the end of each week, then report their progress at the start of the following week's session. Throughout the workshop, participants practice new habits. Leaders of the group encourage participants to achieve small goals that support self-efficacy. During the final week, the group discusses long-term action plans and some of the workshop takeaways participants found most helpful. One retired business leader who participated in the workshop said he had set goals throughout his career and just hadn't thought about doing the same in retirement. He was glad he had taken the workshop—it rekindled a part of him that had been lying dormant. The workshop reminded him that he could build on that momentum now, later in life.

What Doesn't Kill Us

For older adults who may have lived a lifetime of less-than-stellar health habits, it's difficult to imagine how small changes in thoughts and actions over time might lead to better health. Consider the research by Stephen Joseph, a psychologist at the University of Nottingham, whose work with trauma survivors led to writing, *What Doesn't Kill Us: The New Psychology of Posttraumatic Growth*. From his research, Joseph found the experiences of trauma victims more often led to growth than to disorder (Joseph, 2013). He reviewed studies on victims of illness, divorce, assault, bereavement, natural disasters, and other trauma. From hundreds of studies, Joseph found post-traumatic growth is almost always the norm. In other words, Joseph found that what doesn't kill us certainly can make us stronger! I don't want to minimize the pain suffered by the victims in Joseph's research but rather I want to illustrate that the human body can recover and be strengthened, even after bad experiences.

Have you led a charmed life until now? Or have you experienced bad things like illness, divorce, assault, bereavement, and natural disaster? Other trauma? If not trauma, perhaps less painful yet still unfortunate events? Or a series of unfortunate events? According to an article in *Psychology Today*, if you live long enough, you're most likely to experience some significantly stressful event. Someone you love will die. You will get sick or be treated badly. According to the article, "We live in a world filled with catastrophes. Just click on your favorite news website, and you'll see a long list of stomach-churning, tear-jerking stories. The problem with clinging to the mindset that you or someone you know doesn't deserve to experience a certain painful event, that it's unfair, that it shouldn't have happened, is that it increases suffering." How we move past bad experiences is important. When we accept what happened and move past complacency, we reduce suffering. The writer also recommends accepting what has happened to reduce suffering; this acceptance is then validated by actions. Become a volunteer, write a check, or contribute your efforts in other ways (Puff, 2017).

Moving on takes effort. In her book, *Grit*, Angela Duckworth explains why grit—a combination of passion and persistence—correlates with success. Fortunately, like many other positive attributes, grit can be learned, developed, and grown. Despite setbacks and painful events, when you set new goals consider your passions—at any age. Use an *Amaging™ Affirmation* to support them.

What's your One-, Five-, Ten-, or Twenty-year health strategy?

> *"It will never be perfect. Make it work."*
> —Your Life

I mentioned Dr. David Agus's book, *A Short Guide to a Long Life*, in an earlier chapter. Dr. Agus also writes about developing a one-, five-, ten-, and twenty-year health strategy. Think about where you want your health to be in ten years, and then ask yourself, "What can I do differently today to get there?" Agus describes the importance of setting goals, staying focused, and having something to look forward to. He recommends making your own definition of health and then creating your own personal "code of health" along with the rules you will live by to follow your code (Agus, 2014). This code then leads to healthy habits or routines. In appendix 1, I share a fill-in-the-blank tool you can use for both short-term and long-term goals. Your goals may relate to your health strategies or other needs and wants that matter to you.

Recently, this message by an anonymous writer appeared on my Facebook feed, and it gives some small goal examples:

> *Start by doing one push up*
> *Start by drinking one cup of water*
> *Start by paying toward one debt*
> *Start by reading one page*
> *Start by walking one lap*
> *Start by attending one event*
> *Start by writing one paragraph*
> *Start today*
> *Repeat tomorrow*

Imagine how these incremental steps will help you achieve your goals. Notice the key words *start*, *one*, and *repeat*. As you start, make one step initially, and then repeat. Over time, you will not only work toward achieving your goals but you will also build self-efficacy.

Jack Canfield, the *Chicken Soup for the Soul*^R co-author mentioned in the earlier discussion on affirmations, has developed success-coaching principles. In the area of stress and anxiety, some people constantly anticipate the future or relive the past with a "should have" or "could have" attitude. Sound familiar? Many of us are guilty of this at different times in our lives. Canfield gives three recommendations for overcoming obstacles. These three recommendations ring true for me.

As I reviewed these materials while doing research for this book, I smiled a little, thinking I have unknowingly checked off all three while working through difficult situations. This is what Canfield suggests:

- **Lean into it.** Instead of stressing about the issue, take action and keep moving forward. This is how you create momentum. (And I would advocate that this is how you can help create *amaging*^{TM} momentum!)
- **Chunk it down**. Break your bigger goals into smaller, achievable tasks. Start with the first step.
- **Clean up your messes and incompletes.** Look at the different areas of your life, home, and business. What might you have ignored? Left undone? Those unfinished things can create "subconscious stress and anxiety" that may keep you from enjoying life.

Plan Your Day to Build Momentum

One of the best ways to build momentum over time and achieve goals involves planning. Every day. As our age increases, time becomes a more and more precious commodity. Planning becomes more essential. If you struggle with consistently blocking time for what matters most, you may want to try the following method. I'm suggesting the "Top 5

Method," which comes from Sean Ogle, owner of the Location Rebel, a business that helps entrepreneurs find ways to make a living while traveling (Ogle, 2014).

As it turns out, travel and work are hard to do simultaneously. It takes discipline and some strategy to get the job done when you would rather explore new sights. What I like most about Ogle's method is the simplicity. I like to review my Top 5 list at 4:00 p.m. and plan for the next day. Although I don't usually finish work as early as 4:00 p.m., I've found this time of day works for a time-out. I reflect on the day's progress and write things out before my brain is "too fried" to think through the next day's priorities. Then, after pausing for this planning moment, I have a little extra energy to finish a project or start a small one before I'm done working for the day.

Below are the five tasks in the "Top 5 Method." Notice there is a rank-ordering process based on how easy and fun or hard and unpleasant a task may feel:

1. **Something easy or fun** to you start your workday. This way you can "break the productivity ice," and this will help you build momentum quickly.
2. The **hardest thing,** or the least fun thing you want to do on this day. You don't want to put this off until later in the day when you have less energy. Do it now, and the rest of the day will feel more "downhill."
3. The **second hardest** thing. Do you see how this strategy works? Do your least favorite things early.
4. **Something else** that has to get done. This should be something you perceive as easier than numbers two and three on this list.
5. **Something fun.** It does not have to be related to work, or, if you are retired, it would not have to be an obligatory activity like home maintenance, bill paying, decluttering, other paperwork, etc. This might be meeting a friend, going golfing, or going to the gym, for example. Pick an activity you enjoy that has a positive benefit (Ogle, 2014).

Here's an example of how I applied this strategy and prioritized a Saturday morning of working in my home office:

1. Sort a pile of household paperwork I have been neglecting (sorting is easy for me—dealing with it is the hard part).
2. Respond to our family tax accountant about three questions she had as she was preparing our taxes. I'm not sure why, but anything related to taxes usually lands in the "least favorite" category for me!
3. Work on this book for at least ninety minutes without interruption.
4. Edit what I've written.
5. Walk outdoors and listen to a book on tape. The book I'm listening to is also research for writing this book, and in combination with a walk outside on a nice day, it becomes enough of a fun incentive to be the fifth item on my list.

You may have another method, and you may have found another time of day that works better for you. There is not a right or wrong way to plan your day. Consistency matters. By planning your most important things in advance, you can be more intentional about how you focus your energy, and you will find you are putting less energy into schedule-related decisions.

Also, there are a few benefits when you save a fun activity for the end. In this "Top 5 Method," you may find numbers one to four pass more quickly because you have something enjoyable ahead. Number five is an incentive to help you push through. Also, once you knock off four items, if you are feeling good momentum, you certainly can work ahead and do a few more tasks before getting to (and enjoying) number five. When I do this, I will often go back and add these into my list—so I can give myself the extra credit—and I call these tasks 4b., 4c., and so forth! My endorphins appreciate a little boost every time I cross something off the list, so I want to write it down and then cross it off! Also, notice the reframing here—when I get more done than initially planned, I call it "extra credit." This feels better than "super busy" or "overwhelmed" or an "never-ending list."

If you follow this format every day, you will consistently make time for something fun every day—never a bad thing!

If you struggle with consistently planning your day, you may want to use or adapt the *Amaging™ Affirmation* I wrote to support a daily planning habit:

FIGURE 4 *AMAGING™ AFFIRMATION*: BUILDING A HABIT TO PLAN MY DAY

Step 1: What do you really want?

I want to plan my day and include time to work on what is important, not only what is most urgent or most pleasant.

Step 2: What is your growth mindset to support this?

I want to make the most of every day I'm blessed with. To achieve this planning goal, I want to think of day planning as running a marathon, not a sprint.

Step 3: Why do you want it?

Some of the reasons I want to achieve this goal include _____
(list your reasoning, the benefits and positive outcomes related to success).

Step 4: What new hat will you wear?
Describe what type of person you are willing to become.

An overprotective calendar police person. I will be someone who fiercely protects my calendar and is especially inflexible with the appointments I have made relating to my goals.

I will be someone with high self-integrity, honoring the appointments I make with myself. Just as I routinely keep appointments with other people in my life, I will keep the appointments I make with myself to achieve my big goals. Hyper self-aware of my energy, I will be fully present to my own energy levels and manage my energy levels well, so I can work as efficiently and effectively as possible (Miller, 2020).

Step 5: What are you committed to doing? Be specific.

I will only achieve my goals if I consistently put in the time and effort to be successful. I will take some time every day to plan my day. I will start by giving myself twice as much time as I think I'll need for important tasks. I will set aside one- to two-hour sections of time to work on my bigger goals. I will include unstructured time in my calendar for urgent issues and to catch up if I fall behind on my plans. I will include time for fun, exercise, and recreation. I will remember to include time for self-care, including hygiene, nutrition, meditation, exercise, etc. (Soukup, 2019)

Step 6: How will you encourage yourself?

Reinforce your affirmation with one or more inspirational quotes, proverbs, or scripture to build momentum and achieve your goal. Don't skimp on this step!

> *(About day planning)... The reality is that while you've now given yourself a clear road map—or, in modern terms, you've programmed the GPS—you still have to actually drive the car and get yourself to where you want to go. ... You need to make the daily decisions to follow through with your plan and actually do the work.*
>
> —*Ruth Soukup,* Do it Scared

> *Look carefully then how you walk, not as unwise but as wise, making the best use of the time, because the days are evil. Therefore, do not be foolish, but understand what the will of the Lord is.*
>
> —*Ephesians 5:15-17*

Every minute you spend in planning saves ten minutes in execution; this gives you a 1,000 percent return on energy!

—Brian Tracy, author and motivational speaker

A goal without a plan is just a wish.

—Antoine de Saint-Exupéry, writer and pioneering aviator

We have to be purposeful about making sure the big stuff gets done first. We must accept the truth that if we don't take the time to put our long-term goals first, there will never be enough time or energy for our dreams. The obligations of the everyday will always take over.

—Ruth Soukup, Do It Scared

How to Eat an Elephant

According to the World Wildlife Organization, elephants are currently endangered, so I'm not advocating that people eat elephants. "How to eat an elephant? One bite at a time" is a wise maxim to break down a large project into bite-sized pieces. I heard this often early in my career, as my boss at a community hospital used this saying frequently. He had a kind and lighthearted way of helping me reframe a situation to consider the smaller steps to achieve a goal. Whether we were discussing a large fundraising goal, a series of newsletter articles, or a policy change with far-reaching changes, his guidance would usually include this maxim about how to eat an elephant. He didn't want me to get overwhelmed by the magnitude of a project but rather give attention to the more immediate and more doable steps.

There is an instruction book to help break down the complex into the simple. It's titled *Atomic Habits* by James Clear. This is such a brilliant concept! When you think about the definition of *atomic*, these tiny particles have the potential to produce big energy. As Clear discusses in his book, the challenge with tiny advances is they can be so small that they feel insignificant at the time, thus making it hard to stay motivated and stay consistent. Yet many repeated small actions may lead to powerful things. This is a great concept for older adults who want to build *amaging*™ momentum!

Regardless of how many years are behind us, now is a good time to give more attention to breaking bad habits, overcoming negative emotions and self-talk, getting out of our "comfort zone," and setting new goals. One of the key steps in Clear's book is to develop a stronger identity and believe in oneself. This is another good antidote to age bias (see chapter 4). As we age, our own thoughts and today's youth-centered culture may work against us.

7

Thinking with the Enemy

We all know a "glass is half-empty" person, or maybe a few. If the glass is 50 percent filled with water, this person would not see the glass half-*full*, but rather as half-*empty*, and may examine the contents further and determine the water appears to be a tad cloudy, and perhaps a bit too warm or too cold. The "half-empty" person may even find the water has a funny smell to it, and, by the way, did you notice the rim of the glass has an ever-so-tiny chip? Then this same person might suggest drying the glass by hand with a dish towel next time and avoid using the dishwasher for glassware as a way to prevent some of those unsightly water spots…blah, blah, blah.

Do you know someone like this? Maybe that someone is you? It's likely. The human brain is wired to be more pessimistic than optimistic (Alidina, 2015). This theory is called "negativity bias," and this bias supported basic survival when humans were hunters and gatherers. Humans who were extra cautious had a constant eye for danger, and those who scrutinized situations shrewdly were more likely to survive. Researchers have found the human brain gravitates toward more stress and less well-being in three ways:

- overestimating threats
- underestimating opportunities
- underestimating our ability to manage opportunities (Alidina, 2015)

This ability to shrewdly scrutinize may be helpful as hunters and gatherers; however, it can be detrimental when overused—particularly when someone is continually scrutinizing him- or herself.

If this is not enough to convince you to talk nicely to yourself, perhaps the bathroom scale might help convince you to rethink your thoughts. Jean Kristeller, Ph.D., is an advocate for mindful eating; in her book, *The Joy of Half a Cookie*, she describes the importance of mindful eating and mentions the impact of negative self-talk and eating more comfort foods.

> *"Every time you criticize yourself, you strengthen the urge to eat as an escape from the pain of criticism,"* Kristeller says in her book. She advocates for shifting one's mindset from self-criticism to awareness. Mindful eating leads to more awareness and accountability, without self-judgment (Kristeller, 2015).

It is probably no surprise that self-love and self-talk are close cousins. The strength of your loving attitude influences how you talk to yourself. There are ways to love yourself more. In an article, "Top 5 Ways to Get Your Goddess On," the writer shares these tips (Peppler, 2013):

- Bring more playfulness into life. Cultivate things like cooperation, compassion, creativity. Move more. Seek joy.
- Be authentically you. Avoid comparing yourself with others. Be comfortable in your own skin, in the way that you move, hold yourself, and laugh.
- Be warm with others.

- Express yourself creatively. Find a creative outlet—cooking, gardening, music, woodworking, or something else.
- Do more of the things you love. Habitually.

Is there a disconnect between how you talk to others and your self-talk? In Nancy Price's 1987 novel, *Sleeping with the Enemy*, the main character Laura (played by Julia Roberts in the movie) is married to a charming and wealthy businessman who cruelly controls and abuses her—all behind closed doors. Laura's friends and family think she is married to a loving and supportive husband, when in fact she is sleeping with the enemy. Her marriage was all a façade.

I mention this story as a lead-in to the question, "What is your self-talk like?" Are the words in your mind kind and considerate of other people, yet harsh and uncaring toward yourself? Do you criticize yourself more than necessary? Do you talk to yourself like Laura's cruel husband talks to Laura in *Sleeping with the Enemy*, and battling your own internal verbal abuse? Are you thinking with the enemy? Putting on a façade? You may want to use appendix 1 to write your own *Amaging™ Affirmation* to help you improve your self-talk. Or, feel free to use or adapt the *Amaging™ Affirmation* I've written in figure 5 to help you develop more self-compassion.

OPTIMISM CAN BE LEARNED

An important theme in this book is that things can be learned at any age. The *Amaging™ Affirmation* framework supports this learning and helps you identify a growth mindset to propel you forward, your personal "why," the steps you will take to make progress, along with heavy doses of motivation to help you maintain your enthusiasm. It is a myth that optimism is something with which people are either born (perhaps my friend Ginny) or not. Martin Seligman explains this in his book *Learned Optimism*. As a psychology researcher, Seligman studied both helplessness and optimism, and he found that both can be learned. An example of learned optimism is often what happens with victims of domestic violence who may have entered a relationship with great optimism only to have it chip away until it becomes a downward spiral of pessimism, depression, and even illness—in other words, a toxic relationship.

When something bad happens, do you imagine the worst? Do bad events undermine everything you do? Or do you have a sense that whatever happened is manageable—a challenge that can be overcome? Seligman advocates for positive and optimistic mindsets. Optimists do much better academically, they tend to have better health, and they age well (Seligman, 2006). The good news from Seligman is that optimism can be learned. Focusing on positive strengths rather than focusing on negative weaknesses is a key to developing more optimism. In a later book, *Authentic Happiness,* Seligman shares the following five steps (ABCDE) to help develop optimism:

- **Adversity:** Something bad happens.
- **Beliefs:** Examine the beliefs you automatically have or assumptions you make when the adverse event occurs.
- **Consequences of the beliefs:** If you did not change your beliefs, how might this serve you? Or sabotage you?
- **Disputing your belief:** Evaluate and reframe your situation in a more optimistic way.
- **Energization:** Observe the energy return or feelings of hope and empowerment that occur when you successfully challenge your automatic beliefs.

In the *Amaging*™ *Affirmation* framework, there is a pause to reflect and examine mindset in step 2: What is your growth mindset to support this? This aligns with Seligman's belief-related steps; mindset is defined as a belief that orients the way we handle situations. When we decide what to do next, our mindset guides us. As you create your own *Amaging*™ *Affirmations* in step 2, consider how you might reframe your situation in a more optimistic way. Ask yourself how you might shift from a fixed to growth mindset.

Finding the Energy to Overcome Negative Self-Talk

In your own defense, if you find yourself saying unkind words when you talk to yourself, it may be that your energy is running low and self-negativity is a default mode you gravitate toward when you lack energy, when you feel overwhelmed (too busy), or when you feel bored or not stimulated. In her book, *How to Have a Good Day*, Caroline Webb, a management consultant and executive coach, maps out how to set intentions for your day, make the hours go further, make the most of every interaction, leverage your enthusiasm, and in general make the most of every day. She explains how to boost brainpower and start with positive framing. "The trick is to neutralize the sense of threat, so we operate in discovery mode rather than defensive mode," she writes.

Webb suggests assessing recent positive events or imagining the ideal outcome of a project before working on it. In addition to positive framing, Webb outlines some brain-boosting techniques to help you think more clearly (Webb, 2016):

- **Break a complex task down into its parts.** Draw it out, step by step. Allow yourself to focus on one thing at a time and reduce the load on your brain. In retrospect, I realized that I used this technique when writing this book. I created a matrix, and each row has a different subject or chapter, and then I had a column for a related story, scholarly reference, and "why does this matter?" followed by a sample affirmation. Then, as each section was written, I checked it off. This helped prevent overwhelm.
- **Harness your social brain.** Imagine parts of the problem as people! Carry on a pretend conversation with this "person" and walk through the issue by having a conversation with the problem with which you are wrestling.
- Look after what Webb describes as **"smart basics."** This includes removing distractions, doing physical activity, and getting a decent night's sleep.

It may help to remember that as long as you are breathing, there is more right with you than is wrong with you, no matter what you are going through! Does this sound overly optimistic? In another reference book, *The Mindful Way Through Stress*, Shamash Alidina encourages readers to think about what happens in your body when breathing. Your body is nourishing itself with a balanced level of oxygen and then exhaling excess gases. The act of breathing is a miracle, and this miracle happens each time your chest rises and falls.

So, just breathe! Then congratulate yourself for a breath well-done.

When your self-talk is more critical than self-affirming, it can be a stressful way to live. In chapter 12, I share a simple strategy to lean on—a single Bible verse, Philippians 4:8—when struggling with pessimism. Additionally, below is a sample *Amaging™ Affirmation* you may wish to use or adapt to improve self-compassion.

FIGURE 5 *AMAGING™ AFFIRMATION* FOR SELF-COMPASSION

Step 1: What do you really want?

I want my mind to be more self-compassionate.

Step 2: What is your growth mindset to support this?

I believe words matter, especially the words I use when I talk to myself.

Step 3: Why do you want it?

When I am at peace with myself, I will be more comfortable and less anxious with others. I will experience true joy.

Step 4: What new hat will you wear? Describe what type of person you are willing to become.

My own best friend. This means talking to myself as a friend would talk to me.

Step 5: What are you committed to doing?

I will read more about self-compassion and set goals to accomplish it. I will be disciplined to do activities to develop my personal growth. I will take time each day to meditate. I may journal the ways I have been helpful toward others or successful in other ways. I will make a list of my good qualities to refer to when I find myself talking badly to myself.

Step 6: How will you encourage yourself?

Reinforce your affirmation with inspirational quotes, proverbs, or scripture to build momentum and achieve your goal:

> *A moment of self-compassion can change your entire day. A string of such moments can change the course of your life.*
>
> *—Chris Germer*

> *The fruit of the Spirit is love, joy, peace, forbearance, kindness, goodness, faithfulness.*
>
> *—Galatians 5:22*

> *"If you want others to be happy, practice compassion. If you want to be happy, practice compassion.*
>
> *—Dalai Lama*

8
New Tricks for "Old Dogs"

> *Thank God for the privilege of living—*
> *For sharing His earth and His sky—*
> *That a gift so rare as the gift of life*
> *Is given to such as I.*
> —Helen Lowrie Marshall

According to the UK Phrase Finder reference of phrases, "You can't teach an old dog new tricks" is speculated to be among the oldest proverbs in the English language. The phrase has been found in literature dating back to 1534 in John Fitzherbert's book, *The Boke of Husbandry*. Throughout history, this proverb has been repeatedly proven false.

Consider these examples from a collection of later-life learners presented by History.com (Andrews, 2018):

- **Paul Cezanne, painter**, is now considered one of the fathers of modern art. He did not have his first one-man exhibit until 1894, at **age 56**. He went on to produce many masterpieces before dying at **age 67**.

- **Miguel de Cervantes, author**, wrote *Don Quixote* in his **late fifties**. He continued learning the publishing trade, writing and publishing until his death at **age 68**.
- **Julia Child** was a popular **French cook** on television for three decades. She learned to cook **in her forties** and began the television show in 1963, at **age 50**.
- **Ray Kroc** purchased the **McDonald's restaurant** from Richard and Maurice McDonald at **age 53,** in 1961. He then learned the business and transformed McDonald's into a successful fast-food business worth $8 billion at the time of his death nearly two decades later.
- **Laura Ingalls Wilder, author**, was **age 65** when *Little House on the Prairie* was published. She went on to write many more Little House books over the next eleven years.

These are examples of older adults making history later in life. However, the examples listed above are still relatively young!

Here are a few examples of people who learned amazing "new tricks" much later in life:

- **Phyllis Sues, 92,** Los Angeles—learned new music to dance an **Argentine tango** and perform onstage with her dance instructor—in three-inch heels.
- **Nola Ochs, 95,** Kansas—may be the world's oldest **college graduate**, earning a degree in 2007 from Fort Hays State University.
- **Yuichiro Miura, 80,** Japan—looking for a new adventure, he learned to **climb Mount Everest** and scaled it in 2013.

A more recent example is the story of **Tom Capehart, 86, a retired insurance agent** who earned his bachelor's degree from the University of Southern California in 2020 (Schmidt, 2020). During his career, Capehart owned his own life insurance agency with offices throughout southern California, and for more than sixty years he was just two credits short of a bachelor's degree in physical education. Sports were a big deal in Capehart's early years. He had enjoyed competitive sports, and the team camaraderie helped him overcome childhood adversities. Capehart was a four-sport athlete: football, baseball, basketball, and swimming. Then in 1952, during his senior year in high school, he accepted a USC football scholarship.

Unfortunately, a knee injury in his first collegiate game ended his football career. This didn't deter Capehart from loving sports, and he turned his attention to competing with the water polo and the swim team. Unfortunately, his knee injury prevented him from taking the remaining classes that involved boxing, wrestling, and gymnastics.

Capehart moved on. He turned his attention to insurance courses, learning the insurance business, marrying, becoming a father, and raising a family. Years later, Capehart tried to return to finish his degree at USC and found the university no longer offered a physical education degree. Eventually, he found a way to achieve a goal that was so important to him earlier in life.

Fast-forward to 2020: After working with an advisor in the school of education, the university allowed Capehart to earn his diploma by writing his autobiography. He shared a powerful story and was invited to speak at the graduation ceremony as an inspiration to fellow graduates.

No Shortage of New Things to Master

Look to your circle of family, friends, and your community, and it's likely you can add to the list of elders who have achieved remarkable accomplishments. Perhaps you have a feat you have accomplished and can add to this list? Or one you hope to achieve? What *amaging*™ things have you done in your later years? What do you plan to do in the days and weeks ahead?

Consider these examples of what older adults are learning these days:

- New sports such as pickleball. This game combines tennis and ping-pong and is played on a smaller tennis court. (Warning: pickleball may become habit-forming!)
- How to swim or a new swimming stroke.
- Yoga, tai chi, or qigong.
- How to use a computer, tablet, smartphone, smart TV, DVR, video game consoles, and other technologies.
- How to use free weights, resistant bands, circuit training equipment, or other apparatus to build muscle and strength.
- How to grow tomatoes, herbs, flowers, and doing other gardening activities.
- How to sew apparel, quilts, Halloween costumes, doll clothes, household décor, and other items.
- How to use woodworking tools and follow blueprints; how to build and finish furniture, wooden crafts, trim work, decking, and other woodworking projects.
- How to plan a meal; grocery shop; follow a recipe; clean and chop vegetables and fruit; use a stove, food processor, blender, and other kitchen gadgets to cook for oneself or others.
- Much more!

Thanks to the magic of YouTube, Etsy, and other websites with how-to tutorials, today there are many online learning opportunities with step-by-step guides to help people of all ages learn new skills. If online sources are not a good option for you, your local library can likely help fill the void.

This list illustrates some doable feats for most anyone willing to put forth the effort. There is no shortage of new things for older adults to master. Of course, there is often a great shortage of motivation, confidence, and enthusiasm to try and stick with learning or practicing new things until they are mastered or even somewhat accomplished. Small behavior changes, over time, can lead to big improvements. Learning new things can help bring about better health and happiness or just make life easier for an older adult. Notably, a lack of motivation, confidence, or enthusiasm is most certainly a challenge for all ages, not just older adults.

Sometimes modifications may be needed to achieve a new goal. For example, I would like to develop a new biking routine. Yet, in order to do this, I would like to modify the type of bike I am using. On my wish list is an adult tricycle that is lightweight with a practical basket, a not-too-obnoxious horn, a comfortable gel seat, and an all-important rearview mirror. If this tricycle were available in pink or another fun color with a few bling accents, I think that would be pretty neat. And make it electric! I wouldn't use the motor all the time, but it would be a much more enjoyable ride going up hills.

I know how to ride a traditional two-wheel bike, and I do not have a fear of riding a two-wheeler. I also do not aspire to use a new tricycle to train for an Ironman race! I simply think I would enjoy the ride more with a well-blinged adult tricycle with less rigorous balancing effort needed than for a two-wheeler.

It's not uncommon, and likely not considered ageist, to hear someone comment that only young people can learn a new language. Contrary to popular belief, older adults can certainly learn new languages. In case you are wondering how this is feasible, consider a few common methods used to learn a new language:

- Become immersed in the language by traveling.
- Practice it every day.
- Carry a translating dictionary or phone app as a ready reference.
- Watch TV shows or movies in the new language.
- Read and practice writing the language.
- Listen to podcasts or radio shows in the new language.

I've listed only a few of the ways one can learn a new language to illustrate how it can be done, regardless of age. The key is to apply attention and consistent practice.

Why Bother with New Tricks?

> *"If you look at obstacles as a containing fence, they become an excuse for failure. If you look at them as a hurdle, each one strengthens you for the next."*
>
> —Ben Carson

After living five, six, seven, eight, or more decades, it's understandable that you may want to throw your hands in the air and say, "Why bother?" at the thought of starting, learning, adopting, or transitioning to anything new or different. Been there. Done that. I get it.

To answer this age-old "Why bother?" question, I'd like to go back to the growth mindset described in the *Little Engine That Could*. During my work in health-care organization development, I have been honored to work with clinicians to help advance their person-centered communication skills. Some of the key topics we have explored together include empathy, active listening, engaging patients and families in their care plans, hard conversations, and other topics. Whenever possible, during learning activities, the topic of "mindset" has been infused into the discussion. In my role, I would set up the given situation for role-play and then, before starting, pause and brainstorm what a "growth mindset" might be for this situation. Here are a few examples:

- Before talking with an overweight patient about healthy body mass index, a growth mindset might be something like, "Today, I'm planting a seed that will begin to grow for this patient when the time is right," or perhaps, "This patient deals with stress by overeating. I don't want to add more stress with my tone of voice or uncaring words."
- Before talking with a waiting room full of adult children about their aging father, whose health is declining and has little hope for recovery, a growth mindset might be something like, "Emotions may be running high. I am going to do my best to

stay present, stick with my bottom-line message, and repeat it as many times as necessary—with a lot of caring."
- Before telephoning a colleague who I think dropped the ball on something for a patient, a growth mindset might be something like, "I want to describe the specific situation, explain how this impacted my patient, and consider that everyone can learn and grow."

From these activities, clinicians experience taking time out to think about their mindset before a difficult situation. Using a fixed mindset, one's thinking capabilities are limited, and one might consider the weight-loss discussion a lost cause. Why bother? A fixed mindset of thinking the family's emotions will override any patient's preferences might lead to a course of action that is not patient centered. Why bother? Using a fixed mindset, one might think the colleague became busy and we all make mistakes, and therefore one might avoid a difficult phone call all together. Why bother?

The answer to this question is, "Because people's health, your work satisfaction, and the care team's success will sometimes depend on difficult conversations going well."

When we believe there is potential to learn or grow, there is no reason to think a "new trick" isn't worth the time, energy, maybe some discomfort, and likely some great reward, accomplishment, or a little pride at the end. If you catch yourself saying, "Why bother," this may be a red flag that you are stuck in a fixed mindset. After a pause for reflection, you may be able to move toward a growth mindset that can help you forge ahead with success.

My husband is a high school basketball coach, and he has a favorite locker room poster that I think fits well with this idea of learning "new tricks" at any age. Knowledge, hard work, and a positive attitude are important, and of the three, *attitude* is key:

Coincidence?

If:

A	B	C	D	E	F	G	H	I	J	K	L	M
1	2	3	4	5	6	7	8	9	10	11	12	13

N	O	P	Q	R	S	T	U	V	W	X	Y	Z
14	15	16	17	18	19	20	21	22	23	24	25	26

THEN

K	N	O	W	L	E	D	G	E	
11+	14+	15+	23+	12+	5+	4+	7+	5	= 96%

AND

H	A	R	D		W	O	R	K	
8+	1+	18+	4+		23+	15+	18+	11	= 98%

Both are very important, but they fall short of 100%. The maximum value is:

A	T	T	I	T	U	D	E	
1+	20+	20+	9+	20+	21+	4+	5	=100%

BECOMING A MORNING PERSON

Earlier, I shared an example of an affirmation I wrote to help build a writing habit. For five-plus decades of truly disliking the first hour of each day, making my mornings very rushed, I would wait until the last possible minute to jump out of bed, hit the ground running, and start my day. (The exception to this was the years when my daughters were infants to toddlers, and I was able to adopt a better morning habit.)

Yet, to seriously and intentionally write this book and achieve my goal to finish the manuscript and submit it to a publisher, I realized it was time for this *old dog to learn a new trick*! I realized it was time to become a morning person.

I should add that I was able to work on a few goals, not just writing, during my new morning routine. Because I was having trouble drinking the recommended number of ounces of water per day to stay well hydrated, my doctor suggested I drink thirty-two ounces before breakfast. Sounds easy? Try it! I realized I cannot chug water at any time of the day, and especially not in the morning. If I didn't want to skip breakfast (consistently eating breakfast was another goal of mine), I needed to start my thirty-two-ounce water routine at least forty-five minutes to thirty minutes before breakfast. An hour was better. Also, I have experienced on-and-off sciatic nerve pain. I found a few stretching exercises seemed to help. I was committed to maintaining the gain and not sliding back and enduring these shooting pains as a normal part of aging.

This combination of wanting to write, drink more water, and get in a few morning stretching exercises became my much-needed incentive to get an earlier start to my day. To help me overcome my "hitting the snooze button" addiction, I created an affirmation. It helped to read it each morning, and even more helpful was to read it before bedtime.

Here's an example of my morning-person affirmation:

FIGURE 6 AMAGING™ AFFIRMATION TO RISE AND SHINE!

Step 1: What do you really want?

I want to look forward to the morning, wake up, get up, give thanks for a new day, and be productive earlier in the day.

Step 2: What is your growth mindset to support this?

I believe I was not born to be a "snooze-aholic," and I can learn, practice, and develop a habit to wake up earlier.

Step 3: Why do you want it?

I want to make the most of every part of the day, including mornings, for each day remaining in this life.

Step 4: What new hat will you wear? Describe what type of person you are willing to become.

I am committed to becoming a morning person, someone who follows a routine, someone who enjoys a more relaxed and less hurried start to my day.

Step 5: What are you committed to doing?

I will set my alarm each night and put it away from my bed, so I must physically get out of bed to stop the alarm. I will plan my clothes, pack any lunch or snacks, and take any needed steps to prepare for the next day before going to bed. This means I will start getting ready for the next day and for bed before 9:00 p.m. I am committed to less "screen time" in front of the television or computer and more "doing time" to achieve this.

Step 6: How will you encourage yourself?

Reinforce your affirmation with inspirational quotes, proverbs, or scripture to build momentum and achieve your goal.

> *But I will sing of your strength,*
>   *in the morning I will sing of your love;*
> *for you are my fortress,*
>   *my refuge in times of trouble.*
> *You are my strength, I sing praise to you;*
>   *you, God, are my fortress,*
>   *my God on whom I can rely*
>
>   *—Psalm 59:16-17*
> *(Look to God for strength to achieve morning goals;*
>   *sing praise to God in the morning!)*

I am committed to waking up on time tomorrow because 1) Doing so will enable me to develop the discipline I need to succeed in all areas, and 2) I know that how I start each day determines how I create my life because my day is my life.

—Hal Elrod, *from* The Morning Miracle™

The reality is, my mind controls my body, and I really only need as much sleep as I tell myself and choose to believe that I need. Many of the most successful people in history have functioned optimally on (less) sleep, and I cannot allow myself to fall into the limiting belief that sleeping more will somehow improve my life.

—Hal Elrod, *from* The Morning Miracle™

Aging in Reverse?

Imagine how different life might be if we were born old and then each year we lost one year of age. If we aged in reverse. Over time, we would have the wisdom that comes from aging combined with a more youthful physical body. Sounds divine! This concept played out in a screenplay written by Eric Roth called *The Curious Case of Benjamin Button*. The screenplay is an adaptation of F. Scott Fitzgerald's short story with the same title, which was published in 1922.

Benjamin, portrayed by actor Brad Pitt in the 2008 film, was born at age 70 and gets younger at the same rate that everyone else ages. Benjamin's wisdom, the type that comes from years of experience and lessons learned the hard way, was summarized well in a letter written to another character in the film named Caroline, the adult daughter of Daisy, who was Benjamin's love interest in the film:

It's never too late, or in my case too early, to be whoever you want to be. There's no time limit. Start whenever you want. You can change or stay the same. There are no rules to this thing. We can make the best or the worst of it. I hope you make the best of it. I hope you see things that startle you. I hope you feel things you never felt before. I hope you meet people who have a different point of view. I hope you live a life you're proud of, and if you're not, I hope you have the courage to start all over again (Roth, 2008).

Regardless of your age, it's never too late. Be courageous. Live a life you're proud of. Learn new tricks. Start today. For a more visual inspiration, you can watch the scene when actor Brad Pitt writes this letter. Visit YouTube at https://tinyurl.com/ageinreverse.

9

Having Good Friends and Being a Good Friend

I am so blessed to have a good friend of many years. We met on the first day of kindergarten and stayed friends in elementary, middle, and high school. After college, and for many years after that, we fell out of touch and didn't correspond as much. It was my fault; I neglected a valuable friendship. Fast-forward to about fifteen years ago, and we reconnected. My good friend truly "gets me," helping me to look on the bright side of darker situations, making me laugh—a lot—encouraging me to try new things, and just listening when I ramble on. On my birthday last year, she gave me the nicest card, which talked about how I remember the little things that mean so much to others: "You're someone with a special way of bringing on the sunshine and making others' hearts a little lighter—and thanks to you, those little things add up to quite a lot…" I love and value all of my friends, and I especially value this dear friend whom I've known since the first day of public school, who affirms me, strengthens me, and who strengthens our friendship. She is also quite *amaging*^{TM}, by the way!

Friendships are important throughout our life, and recent research shows that friendships have a bigger impact on our health and well-being as we age, according to an article published by AARP (Hayes, Kim, 2017). In a study conducted at Michigan State University with a sample size of approximately 280,000 (this is a very large sample size) researchers found a link between "valuing friendships" and functioning better among older adults. In the same study, "valuing familial relationships" had a static influence on health and well-being for all ages. While family relationships are vital, they didn't prove to have as powerful an impact as friendships. Researchers speculate that family relationships will often include some type of a caregiving obligation. Older adults reported friendships were linked with joy.

While researching this book, I asked some older adults about their personal and their loved ones' struggles with growing old. One woman in her sixties talked about her mother's challenges with loneliness:

> *Friends were also important. Because she lived longer (into her nineties), her friends passed before her. She was one who wanted to provide care for others, like helping them change their bandages or put in their eye drops. Then, it was frustrating for her when she could not take care of others. This made her more depressed when she got older. When she was younger, she used to help others. Then, as she got older, she was in the opposite position of a caregiving role. When some of her siblings and close friends died, she felt like, "I just don't have anyone."*

Another woman with whom I spoke while researching this book also emphasized the importance of friendship, especially after she retired:

> *Although I am pretty comfortable being alone, I find that I do need to make a conscious effort to schedule time with friends on a regular basis. For me, it is about the special connections that bring joy and satisfaction; that is, simply being with another person or a group to socialize isn't sufficient. There needs to be a connection.*

This need for connection is not uncommon, and loneliness is a big deal. The American Psychological Association published a report in 2017 titled "Advancing Social Connection as a Public Health Priority" (Holt-Lunstad, 2017). The article defined the problem and summarized the scope and severity of loneliness.

Loneliness is a multifactorial problem that can include having too few relationships, lacking interactions or support, facing being alone, experiencing strained relationships, and other issues under the umbrella theme of "lacking social connections." The article described this lack of social connectedness as an urgent and severe issue that is also related to economic losses. The urgency is due to the rapid increase in the incidence of loneliness, which may be attributed to a decline in volunteerism, declining religious affiliations, and an aging population (which is more likely to experience loneliness). The severity of the situation is due to the early death rates associated with a lack of social connections.

When compared with other serious health conditions like obesity, inactivity, and smoking, the prevalence of loneliness is far greater. The article recommends more research be done on the costs associated with loneliness. In the few studies cited that evaluated health-care costs and social support, researchers found better treatment outcomes and lower medical costs when test subjects had better social connections (Holt-Lunstad, 2017).

According to the Mayo Clinic, friends can help you improve your health. Friends are important to help you celebrate the good times and to help you cope with the stressful times. Here's what Mayo Clinic's healthy lifestyle tips say friendship will do for you:

- increase your sense of belonging and purpose
- boost your happiness and reduce your stress
- improve your self-confidence and self-worth
- help you cope with traumas, such as divorce, serious illness, job loss, or the death of a loved one

- encourage you to change or avoid unhealthy lifestyle habits, such as excessive drinking or lack of exercise

The article goes on to say it's important to have good friends and to be a good friend. Here are some ways to nurture friendships, according to the Mayo Clinic article:

- be kind
- listen well
- open up (be willing to share some personal experiences)
- show that you can be trusted (be responsible, reliable, dependable, and keep private information private)
- make yourself available (spend time together and check in on each other between visits).

Sometimes as Age Increases, Friendships Decrease

Unfortunately, each year, when the number of birthday candles has gone up, you may find the number of friends in your life has gone down. Usually this is not intentional. Friendships can be lost when older adults make life-changing decisions to move closer to their family, to warmer climates, or to downsize. Friendships may diminish when a friend's health declines and he or she becomes less active or requires institutional care, or when a friend dies. Often with retirement, a person loses the close friendships and relationships that formed from working outside the home. Over time, as friendships are *unintentionally* lost, older adults need to take *intentional* steps to connect with remaining friends and make new friends.

There are some friendship norms described in *Generations*, the journal published by the American Society on Aging. These norms include mutual respect and trust, companionship, mutual support, and a tendency to befriend others who are similar to us. Some friendships—like the relationship I mentioned earlier with my childhood friend—can start early in life and endure for a lifetime. In contrast, as life's circumstances change at any time in life, people are able to acquire new friends. This is normally influenced by personality, outlook, and choice. One benefit of having more time during retirement is the discretion to choose which friends with whom to spend time, which distance friends with whom to stay in touch, and which ones to let fade. (Bliezner, 2014) (Qualls, 2014)

As important as good friendships are to our well-being, it should be noted that problematic friendships can potentially interfere with our health. There may be some value in letting a friendship fade. Unhealthy friendships can damage health. "If friends do not encourage each other to comply with diet, exercise, medication, or other health-related recommendations, if they offer unsolicited and unhelpful advice, if they are self-centered and cannot reciprocate social and emotional support, they are likely to foster psychological distress and diminish health rather than provide the kind of support that sustains general well-being," the author writes (Bliezner, 2014).

STAYING IN TOUCH ACROSS THE MILES

Earlier in my career, I was fortunate to lead a healthy aging program and host a monthly event for older adults for learning and sharing. We reviewed "Blue Zones" research and discussed the attributes of those who live in Blue Zones throughout the world. Blue Zones are where people tend to live longer lives, areas where a higher percent of the population reaches age 100 or greater. A key characteristic in Blue Zones is the support network of friends and family. As we talked about this in our healthy aging group, I led a mini brainstorming session around the question, "How do you stay connected with loved ones?" It's a simple question, but the responses were challenging. There are many obstacles, particularly the geographic distance between loved ones who may move away over the years for work and other reasons. We spent time on this question to help each other think of new and different ways to stay connected. Some of the ideas shared included phone calls, writing letters, sending greeting cards, taking vacations together, using Facebook or other social media, emailing, attending the grandchildren's sporting events, etc.

We learned there is no right or wrong way to stay connected with friends and loved ones. Just proactively make the effort.

Loneliness: A Public Health Issue

Friendships are important—so important that loneliness is considered a public health issue. Researchers have found loneliness and weak social connections are associated with a reduction in lifespan similar to that caused by smoking fifteen cigarettes a day (Schulze, 2018). This impact on lifespan was found to be more significant than obesity. Researchers have discovered that connecting with other people provides a sense of safety and security that lessens the fight-or-flight stress state and lowers perceptions of loneliness. In a 2015 article published by the American Public Health Association, the impact of loneliness on healthcare utilization for older adults was explored (Gerst-Emerson, 2015). Researchers looked at the long-term impact of health care use among community-dwelling elders. While they did not find a relationship between loneliness and hospitalizations, there was a link with physician clinic visits. Those who were lonely were less likely to visit their primary care provider for preventive care, chronic disease management, and for other health concerns.

Friends can help you enjoy life more and obtain a sense of well-being. Intuitively, it makes sense that participating in an uplifting conversation with someone that influences feelings of hope and joy early in a day may lead to more physical activity or healthy food choices later that same day. Through research, healthy relationships have been linked to better blood pressure, heart rate, cholesterol levels, better compliance with health and medication regimens, a greater sense of meaning in life, a stronger sense of purpose, and other positive factors (Qualls, 2014).

Unfortunately, a lack of friendships has been found to have the opposite impact on health. Researchers have found that loneliness increases the risk for early death by 45 percent (Ferrari, 2017). Loneliness is linked to a weakened immune system, higher blood pressure, and a greater risk for heart attacks and strokes. Sara Honn Qualls is a professor of psychology, a director of the Gerontology Center at the University of Colorado, Colorado Springs, and a passionate advocate for the physical and mental well-being of older adults. She writes:

> *Friends journey with us, motivate us, or drag us away from good health. Family members care for each other across the lifespan, with acceleration for periods in later life. Every aging person, or provider of services to aging persons, needs to understand the linkage between good relationships and excellent health.*

In the Blue Zones research I mentioned earlier in this book, social connectedness was linked to the longest living people on the planet. Blue Zones researchers studied demographics across the globe looking for the longest-living humans; then, they sent researchers to uncover the "secrets of long life" (Buettner, 2012). Not surprisingly, having other people around you who care about you was a key lesson shared in the Blue Zones geographical areas where the highest percentages of the population were age 100 or more.

With these connections, life is more worthwhile and days are more meaningful, according to the Blue Zones researcher and author, Dan Buettner. He shares the following tips to build your inner circle within your personal Blue Zone:

- **Identify your inner circle**. Who reinforces good habits? Challenges you mentally? Is reliable in times of need?

- **Be likeable**. When researching centenarians for his book, Buettner said there was not a grumpy person in the bunch. Likeable older adults are more likely to have social connections, visitors, and caring caregivers.
- **Create time together**. Take a look at your calendar. Are you spending at least thirty minutes per day with someone in your inner circle? Buettner said his research has shown the investment in time will pay back in added years lived—a great reward.

When I ask people about their struggles with growing old, one story stands out for me. A woman in her middle fifties described how socialization had become an issue for her aging mother:

> *For my mother, I can see that due to hearing loss and a bad back (also a bit of depression due to the pain), she isolated herself, and we now have dementia starting. I think if she had made more friends, she would have held off dementia.*

Her mother's struggles have motivated her to do more to prevent future dementia and other health problems by eating healthy, physical exercising, doing daily puzzles, and exercising good dental hygiene.

It's Not Too Late to Make Friends

It is never too late in life to build new friendships or reconnect with old friends. The effort you devote toward friendships can result in better health and better well-being throughout this phase of life's journey. Also, investing time and resources in friendship is most beneficial when the friendships inspire you to stay healthy and do healthy activities together (Ehrenfeld, 2017). I visit an online forum that shares challenges, tips, and encouragement with each other. Another member recently posed the question, "How does one make friends?" This was a great question that sparked many impromptu suggestions. Here are some of the ideas offered by this caring online community:

- **Find activities** you enjoy that include others, like taking a yoga class or joining a canoe team. When you find others who enjoy similar activities, you may find you have more in common in other ways as well. Look for events, classes, church programs, choirs, activities, workshops, book clubs, and volunteer opportunities with other people. It's better to take action than to simply read about it.
- Consider joining a Toastmasters club (advocating leadership and better overall communication), gym classes, running groups, short courses focused on hobbies, etc. It will be a little scary when you first step outside your comfort zone, but it will be well worth it.
- **Pray** for friendship! It works!
- **Practice**. Don't give up on yourself.
- Make up **calling cards** at a print shop. Pass them out as you meet people at the gym or when you volunteer or go to the theater. Ask for a coffee date!
- **Smile**. Say hello. Be open to conversation. Complement people. Offer to help. Show an interest in others.
- **Talk less**. Listen more.
- **Don't** look for people who are **just like you**. Be willing to care about someone else's life and invest your time in getting to know them.
- **Join** an adult tap dance class.
- Learn to **love yourself first**. Then they'll come to you. Be yourself.
- Find ways to perform **small acts of kindness** for other people.
- **Shut off your phone** and seek out face-to-face conversation.
- **Read** materials written by Michele Peppler, author of *Be the Queen*. She shares information on how to "create your tribe"

and find deeper connections with likeminded souls. Read *How to Win Friends and Influence People*, by Dale Carnegie. (This book was recommended by multiple followers in the online comments.)

Other books on friendship building that were recommended include the following list:

- *Tell Me More* by Kelly Corrigan
- *Text Me When You Get Home* by Kayleen Schaefer
- *Frientimacy* by Shasta Nelson
- *How to Talk to Anyone—92 Little Tricks for Big Success in Relationships* by Leil Lowndes

As you contemplate action plans for your personal growth, consider setting goals for yourself that will move you away from isolation and grow your inner circle. You may want to take a first step by going to the library in the next seven days to check out one of the above books, or call your local volunteer center or senior center to ask about volunteer opportunities and upcoming classes or events of interest.

Take small steps each week until you reach your friendship goals. Chapter 6 includes more on action planning, an important self-management tool.

A High Friendship Bar

Imagine what it might be like to have 11,000 friends in your lifetime. I am not talking about friends on social media. I'm talking about those friends you spend face-to-face time with, chat with on the phone, or perhaps send a handwritten note card, birthday, or holiday card to on a routine basis. Yes, eleven thousand is an amazing achievement. If you do the math, this would mean adding 110 friends per year or roughly 2.1 new friends per week, every week of your life, including your first year of life before you learned to walk or talk—and that's if you live to be 100. Sound impossible? It's not. It has been done, and it didn't take 100 years—only 67.

It happened during the lifetime of the late Jeff Krause from my hometown in Wisconsin. Quoting from his published obituary:

> *The circle of friends Jeff leaves behind is broad and far reaching. Jeff's name could be in Webster's dictionary defining the word friendship. His humbleness, sincerity, generosity, and care for others never faltered...Jeff always made the time to talk to people, inquiring about family, situations, or whatever happened to be going on in that person's life. Jeff had a wonderfully dry sense of humor and laughed easily...He had warmth and pureness of heart which he willingly shared with all he knew.*

This obituary so accurately described an incredibly gifted person, who I was fortunate to know during my formative high school years. Jeff Krause was my choir director and a friend. I was able to attend his funeral, where his best friend delivered a heartfelt eulogy and described how many lives were made better by knowing Jeff. The eulogist said that while living, Jeff thought his passing would be a mere blimp on the radars of his acquaintances. Jeff certainly underestimated his value to others. At his funeral, the large church was filled to capacity, including an ad hoc alumni choir of former students singing with deep regard for their late, great "Maestro" and friend.

As the eulogist described, Jeff understood that students don't care how much you know until they know how much you care. Four decades after my high school graduation, I still remember feeling like I had a teacher who cared when I walked into his classroom.

Those whom God placed in Jeff's life were blessed to learn Jeff had a talent and love for music that was upstaged by his friend-making talent. Notably, the 11,000 number of friends is a low estimate, counting only the students Jeff taught during his years as a music teacher. In addition to those students who considered Jeff a friend, he was a friend to his family, colleagues, neighbors, and others.

I should add Jeff's friendships were *not* fostered on social media by posting messages, wishing people happy birthday, happy anniversary, and "liking" photos or posts. His friendships weren't virtual. He practiced friendship the old-fashioned way: in person, on the phone, through cards and letters.

So, my friends, the bar has been set high by Jeff Krause. If you think 11,000 friends in a lifetime is not practical for your current situation, then set a goal for a lower number. Set a goal to proactively build your inner circle of friends. Be more like Jeff Krause. You will reach your goal, and your life will be blessed beyond measure. An affirmation you may want to use or adapt to help you reach your friendship goals follows. In step 6, I've included the lyrics from "Seasons of Love," a song sung by the alumni choir and a song that Jeff requested for his memorial service:

FIGURE 7 AMAGING™ AFFIRMATION ON FRIENDSHIP

Step 1: What do you really want?

I want to be a good friend and have good friends.

Step 2: What is your growth mindset to support this?

I believe there are things I can proactively do to avoid loneliness and isolation.

Step 3: Why do you want it?

I want to increase my friendships to improve my well-being and my physical health, and to add more joy to my days.

Step 4: What new hat will you wear? Describe what type of person you are willing to become.

I am committed to reassess my inner "friendship quotient" and identify areas for improvement. Am I a person with integrity? This includes being trustworthy, honest, dependable, loyal, and more trusting of others. Are my behaviors in these areas consistent? Am I as caring as I could be with others? Caring people are empathetic, nonjudgmental, good listeners, and helpful. Am I generally likeable? Someone who is likeable is pleasant and generally fun to be with, and has self-confidence and a sense of humor.

Step 5: What are you committed to doing?

I'm committed to *avoid* activities that might be done by a loner, in solitary or generally by myself, as a rule. Instead, I will look for opportunities with others. I'll attend community events, volunteer, or go to church or faith functions. If I am invited to an event, I will accept the invitation whenever possible. Similarly, I will look for opportunities to invite other people to attend events with me. I will record, remember, and help celebrate birthdays and other special occasions involving my friends.

Step 6: How will you encourage yourself?

Reinforce your affirmation with inspirational quotes, proverbs, or scripture to build momentum and achieve your goal:

> *Walking with a friend in the dark is better than walking alone in the light.*
>
> —Helen Keller

> *"Dear George: Remember no man is a failure who has friends.*
>
> — It's a Wonderful Life

> *I know it is wet and the sun is not sunny, but we can have lots of good fun that is funny.*
>
> —Dr. Seuss, The Cat in the Hat

525,600 minutes
525,000 moments so dear
525,600 minutes
How do you measure, measure a year?
In daylights, in sunsets, in midnights, in cups of coffee
In inches, in miles, in laughter, in strife
In 525,600 minutes
How do you measure a year in the life?
How about love? ...
Measure in love
Seasons of love

—Lyrics from "Seasons of Love" by Jonathan Larson,
from the Broadway musical Rent

10

Better Fitness While Growing Old

While I did research for this book, I asked older adults about their biggest problems with growing older. One woman shared the following:

> *I think the big thing I have struggled with and some friends is the slower metabolism and gaining weight that is such a struggle to lose or keep off. It goes on so easy, but not off! I think the muscle loss that we incur is a big piece of it, but how do you not allow that, or what or when do you need to start working on this before it becomes an issue? ...I'm trying to work on building muscle back up since that is what seems to deteriorate over time.*

Her interest and willingness to gain muscle and retain physical fitness is *amazing*™! So often with our generation, as with our parents' and grandparents' generation, we are less interested in a lifestyle change than we are interested in a quick fix. As a rule, we are generations of people who willingly accept a pill when prescribed. Think about the last time a doctor, nurse practitioner, or physician assistant prescribed a medication for you. Did you ask any of these questions?

- Are there any nondrug alternatives?
- What are common side effects?
- Is this drug-habit forming?
- How or when will it work?
- How will it interact with other pill(s) I'm taking?

Did you ask any questions at all? If you are like most people, you did not. I have talked with pharmacists about this, and they say consumers usually do not ask questions about their medications. I would speculate this is not because people lack curiosity but rather because people (myself included) just *think* what the provider is prescribing will usually work and will help us heal or feel better—no questions asked.

Like a medication, if your health-care team prescribes increased physical activity or exercise, would you accept of it? Do you just *think* that what the provider prescribes will help you heal or feel better—no questions asked? Or do you generally *think* more physical activity will not work for you? Do you usually *think* a prescription for better nutrition will not work for you? Why do we *think* pills will work, but not nutrition? Not exercise? Not meditation? Not stress management?

The late C. Everett Koop, MD, former surgeon general, once said, "Drugs don't work for 100 percent of the people who don't take them." Koop was talking about complex problems that happen when people do not take medications as prescribed (Brody, 2017). Similarly, wellness recommendations do not work for 100 percent of people who do not participate. Exercise is medicine! Healthy foods, particularly vegetables and fruits, are medicine! Of course, it's important to talk with your provider about your medications and to adhere to what is prescribed.

Do you see value in adhering to those nonpharmaceutical prescriptions from your health-care team? This might include prescriptions like walking more for arthritis; eating less sugar for weight loss; using heat or ice for comfort; or using diversions like music, reading, or socializing for pain relief. Just as you trust the pill prescriptions, ask yourself if you can reframe your thinking to trust the nonpill prescriptions.

Sometimes the perception that it's too late in life to make big lifestyle changes stands like a barrier for older adults. A lifetime of unhealthy habits may have resulted in poor health, such as a high body mass index, high cholesterol, poor blood sugar levels, a chronic or ongoing health problem, or multiple ongoing health problems. Having one or more chronic conditions is not uncommon for older adults and may make you feel like your situation is hopeless. Everyday stress without health problems is difficult enough; those with chronic health problems must deal with added stressors like pain or discomfort, time needed to cope with a health condition, new limitations in activities, and financial pressure due to health-care costs. All of these things add up to more frustration, more confusion, and likely more isolation (Madell, 2016).

Because chronic conditions are ongoing and cannot be cured, those who have them need to figure out how to manage the day-to-day problems associated with the conditions.

At age 77, after smoking cigarettes daily for sixty years, my mother stopped smoking. She did this cold turkey after multiple practice attempts to quit. Imagine how difficult this must have been for someone who is widowed, has limited social interactions, and has used cigarettes as a source of comfort and relaxation for decades? When I asked how she was able to make this change after smoking for so long, she said, "I prayed for it when I said my prayers at night, for a long time. God helped me do it."

Her quitting was influenced by her daughter-in-law's (my sister-in-law's) cancer diagnosis. When she first quit, my mother found she chewed more gum, put more puzzles together, and looked for other ways to occupy her time. Fast-forward thirteen-plus years after quitting, and, fortunately, it has stuck (and my sister-in-law is cancer-free)!

When I ask my mother if she misses smoking, she says not really. She's moved on in life. Even though she smoked daily for all those years, she does not miss it. "I don't feel like something else is driving me. I feel free," she said. I love this example of making a change later in life that brings about a better quality of life.

One of the best justifications for improving any lifestyle habit, eating healthier, or being more active—at any age—comes from holy scripture. The Bible reminds us to treat our bodies as if they were precious gifts from God. According to 1 Corinthians, chapter 6, "Do you not know that your body is a temple of the Holy Spirit, who is in you, whom you have received from God? You are not your own; you were bought at a price. Therefore, honor God with your body."

Think back in time to your most memorable Christmas or birthday gifts. Which ones were the most meaningful? Which gifts do you take care of to this day and try to keep in pristine condition? Which of your most prized gifts do you polish, dust, or clean? Wouldn't healthy habits be much easier to adhere to if we adopted a new mindset regarding our own bodies? If we treated our bodies as very precious and special gifts that we want to keep in good working order and protect from harm?

At age 32, Joseph C. Piscatella remembers feeling discomfort in his chest while playing tennis, so he went to the doctor. Two days later he had emergency bypass surgery to correct a 95 percent blockage of his coronary arteries. The prognosis was not good, yet he beat the odds and is still living at the time I'm writing this book, at age 65. Piscatella has written many books on heart health, including, *Positive Mind, Healthy Heart!* He's an advocate for finding ways each day to motivate and inspire healthier habits:

> *It would be great if simply knowing how to live a healthy way could make it happen. We'd be a nation of fit people! But it doesn't work that way. To move from knowing to doing, you need motivation. That's why every day I look for people's stories and sayings to inspire me and keep me on track.*

Piscatella tells the story of a man who didn't have time to exercise on Monday, had a heart attack on Tuesday, and then on Wednesday realized he'd have no problem fitting exercise into his daily routine! Don't wait until your health declines further. It's a lot more fun to exercise for prevention than for rehab. Consider why you want to make a change in your life and then consider the person you are willing to become in order to get there.

Write and use an affirmation at least once daily to keep yourself on the exercise track. Here's an example of an *Amaging™ Affirmation* to build a daily routine. You may want to use this one or adapt it to help you achieve a fitness goal.

FIGURE 8 *AMAGING™ AFFIRMATION* TO MOVE MORE

Step 1: What do you really want?

To develop a habit to exercise or be more active every day.

Step 2: What is your growth mindset to support this?

I believe consistency matters, and I can learn to find the time and energy that's needed.

Step 3: Why do you want it?

By being more physically active, I can reduce the risk of premature death, coronary heart disease, high blood pressure, stroke, metabolic syndrome, type 2 diabetes, falling, and other health problems.

Step 4: What new hat will you wear? Describe what type of person you are willing to become.

An active participant in life, someone who participates in activities and does less watching from a chair or sofa. A good planner. A fervent scheduler who adjusts my calendar as needed to make more time for physical activities. Someone who can bounce back on day two after missing a day of exercise.

Step 5: What are you committed to doing?

Track and record my minutes, miles, laps, or take other measures to monitor my progress over time. Make physical activity a priority, which means giving laser focus to how I manage my time each day. Monitor my emotions, so I truly know when a physical activity brings me joy; then do more of that!

Step 6: How will you encourage yourself?

Reinforce your affirmation with inspirational quotes, proverbs, or scripture to build momentum and achieve your goal:

> *Honor God with your body.*
>
> *—1 Corinthians 6*

> *No matter how slow you go, you're still lapping everybody on the couch."*
>
> *—Elite Daily*

> *"Exercise more. Soon, it's going to feel amazing."*
>
> *—Anonymous*

IF YOU AREN'T DEAD YET, DON'T GIVE UP

I had the privilege of listening to Bevan K. Baker, former commissioner of health for the City of Milwaukee, who spoke at a health-care conference. Baker shared how the Navy SEAL motto "If you aren't dead yet, then don't give up" was an inspiration for his work with the Milwaukee Health Department, the largest health department in Wisconsin, an academic facility with multiple outpatient health centers. As difficult as any of his department's goals were to achieve, Baker felt they could not compare with the hardships, stamina, and rigorous training required of Navy SEALs (Baker, 2017).

I was inspired to do a little research on Navy SEALs, and I learned that to be considered as a Navy SEAL enlisted recruit you need to be able to swim five hundred yards (twenty lengths of a twenty-five-yard pool) in at least twelve minutes and thirty seconds. You have to be able do fifty push-ups, fifty sit-ups, and at least ten pull-ups. You also need to be able to run one-and-a-half miles in under ten minutes and thirty seconds. These are the minimum requirements. For Navy SEAL *officers*, the bar is set higher.

How do future Navy SEAL recruits achieve these goals? The Navy encourages a long-term approach with gradual progress over several months, rather than cramming in workouts for more instant, but short-lived results. According to its website, the Navy recommends the best track to become a Navy SEAL is to *decide* that quitting is not an option, regardless of how challenging the task. The Navy says making this decision increases the likelihood of becoming a Navy SEAL. (U.S. Navy, n.d.)

I would advocate that there are some important lessons older adults can learn from Navy SEALs:

- When goals are incredibly difficult, plan for gradual and incremental progress over several months.
- Setting small daily goals will help you improve things.
- Make a decision not to quit.
- If you are not dead yet, then don't give up!

Of course, becoming a Navy SEAL is *not* likely a goal for most of us. Still, we may want to become more physically active. Physical activity is a "strong protective factor from premature mortality" (Sallis, 2015). In other words, physical activity helps you live longer! Many ongoing diseases and mental health problems, including dementia, are linked to inactivity.

Unlike our great-grandparents, today we drive to a grocery store and garden less, we have more desk jobs and less manual laborers, and we drive or ride in vehicles instead of walking or biking. We enjoy spectator sports, binging TV series and movies, and choose to watch others be active as a form of entertainment. Due to this cultural shift, physical *in*activity is a leading cause of death in the United States. Conversely, researchers have found that physical activity positively affects many major diseases and conditions (Sallis, 2015). Results of a large-scale literature review published by the Agency for Healthcare Research and Quality shows physical activity can reduce the risk of premature death, coronary heart disease, high blood pressure, stroke, metabolic syndrome, type 2 diabetes, breast cancer, colon cancer, depression, falling down, and other health problems. At age 50, an adult who becomes active can add 1.3 to 3.7 years of life (Sallis, 2015).

This may seem like a short amount of time when compared to a lifetime, but think about all you could accomplish with an added 16 to 44 months of life! That's 480 to 1,320 more days, or 11,520 to 31,680 more hours! You might use that time to hold a new grandchild. Teach a teenager how to manage money wisely. Celebrate a loved one's college graduation. Help a neighbor organize a collection of family photos. Help a relative struggling with dementia. Hike a mountain trail. Visit monuments in Washington, DC. Learn to line dance. Finish your bucket list. Start a new bucket list. Whatever it is you want to do, you'll have more time to do it. That's a gift you can give yourself simply by being more physically active.

Moving More

When setting a new physical fitness goal, it is important for older adults to approach physical activity and exercise like a rock climber—safety first and one step at a time. An experienced rock climber looks for a safe next step before making a move. One misstep can be tragic for a rock climber. Safety is very important, not only for rock climbers, but in every sport or activity. As an older adult, it's important to listen to your doctor and your body; do not move ahead until you feel safe. Then do so one step at a time.

For example, if your lifestyle is currently sedentary, and your goal is to walk a one-mile path along the river at your city park, then start slowly. You might set a goal to walk for five minutes before breakfast and five minutes after lunch for three days this week. If you achieve this goal, then you might choose to increase your walking time to seven minutes or stay at five minutes and increase to four days per week. Over several weeks—and only when it feels safe to you—you might up your goals of walking time and frequency until the park path goal is achievable.

By the time we become older adults, we know it's important to be more physically active; however, for many of us, there's something stopping us from moving more. What is one of the key differences between active and inactive older adults? The answer to this question was the focus of a study reported in the *Journal of Aging Studies* (Franke, 2013). In an article titled, "The Secrets of Highly Active Older Adults," researchers discussed the secret to active older adults.

The answer is resourcefulness—a personal trait that relies on self-efficacy, self-control, and adaptability. Researchers found people's environments were important, but resourcefulness was the primary contributor. Oxford Dictionary defines resourcefulness as the ability to find quick and clever ways to overcome difficulties.

Below is an affirmation you may want to use or adapt to help you become more resourceful.

FIGURE 9 ELASTICITY FOR THE SOUL: RESOURCEFULNESS AFFIRMATION

Step 1: What do you really want?

To be resourceful and resilient, able to bounce back after difficulties, learn from them and move forward.

Step 2: What is your growth mindset to support this?

When I'm stuck, I can learn and find ways to get unstuck.

Step 3: Why do you want it?

I want to do my best until I take my last breath. I want to be challenged by difficulties, not paralyzed by them. I want to consider the side effects of bad situations as temporary, not permanent. I want to contain problems, so they do not become pervasive.

Step 4: What new hat will you wear? Describe what type of person you are willing to become.

Adaptable, flexible, and willing to adapt in ways I might not have before. A good historian—someone who learns from my past, so I can adjust and move forward. Courageous—or at least someone who takes even tiny steps with valiant courage. A good self-manager—monitoring my faith, friendships, nutrition, exercise, sleep, and any areas I want to work on for personal growth.

Step 5: What are you committed to doing?

Breathe! When my emotions are running high, I'm committed to taking a few seconds to pause, take a deep breath, and figure out my next steps. I will use visualization to picture myself handling a situation calmly and rationally. I will look for silver linings and when something bad happens, I will try to list a few positives about what happened—or even just a tiny one. I will ask questions and avoid making assumptions. I will practice forgiveness and let go of resentment and grudges *for my own sake*. I will be kind. I will laugh more.

Step 6: How will you encourage yourself?

Reinforce your affirmation with inspirational quotes, proverbs, or scripture to build momentum and achieve your goal.

You gotta shake your brains, figure it out
There's no need to scream or shout
You gotta work that thing you've got upstairs
You gotta activate what's under your hair

—Red and Kathy Grammer

Success and failure come and go, but don't let them define you. It's who you are that matters.

—Kamal Ravikant, Live Your Truth

The human capacity for burden is like bamboo, far more flexible than you'd ever believe at first glance.

—Jodi Picoult, My Sister's Keeper

Everything can change in a heartbeat; it can slip away in an instant. Everything you trust and treasure, whatever brings you comfort, comes at a terrible cost. Health is temporary; money disappears…So, when the moment comes, and everything you depend on changes… must disaster follow? Or will you—somehow—adapt?

—Margaret Overton

11

Better Food Habits While Growing Old

When doing research for this book, I asked a long-term registered nurse and friend about **the problems associated with aging**. She said that older adults often struggle with **healthy body weight** and **physical inactivity**:

> The effects of not eating healthily or overindulging paired with not being physically active enough routinely sets the stage for negatively affecting all the major organs as well as the spine and joints. A cycle that is nearly impossible to break is sometimes the result. Excess weight causes pain and is too much to carry around, but the person gets exhausted and depressed trying and failing to exercise, and ends up eating more and sitting around more. As we age, our metabolism changes, and we need even less food to function. If we don't have control of our weight now, we must get control while we still can, or we may develop diabetes, hyperlipidemia, hypertension, fatty liver, joint pain and replacements, cardiac and vascular problems, and the list

goes on...Like my doctor said to me, it's all about what you put in your mouth.

This nurse described the nearly impossible cycle of poor nutrition and inactivity that so often leads to health problems. The struggle is real. Yet, there are steps we can take at any age to support a healthier body.

In his book, *A Short Guide to a Long Life* (Agus, 2014), Dr. Agus talks about the importance of eating "real food." He recommends looking for foods that do not come with the FDA-approved nutrition fact label. "Steer clear of those aisles lined with boxes and bottles and other food imposters that come in pretty packages," Agus says. He also recommends we eat foods in season because if food is shipped from too great a distance, it may have been picked before it fully ripened, with less time to develop optimal vitamins and minerals. An exception would be frozen fruits and vegetables. If you can't purchase truly fresh produce from a nearby farm, Agus recommends the freezer section at the grocery store, looking for "flash-frozen" foods that are picked when they're ripe, at peak nutritional value, and then frozen.

Some of Agus's other nutrition tips include cooking your own food, moderating food portions, eating with other people, avoiding snacks, and allowing yourself to get hungry between meals.

In this chapter, I'm focusing on two areas related to nutrition: reducing sugar and portion sizes. Throughout my career, clinicians I've worked with have emphasized that food is medicine, and the type of foods we eat matter. However, which specific foods are best for you is a conversation you should have in a clinic exam room with your primary care provider or another specialist. Or experiment by trial and error to determine what foods help or hinder any symptoms you are experiencing. I am assuming that less added sugar and smaller portion sizes are beneficial in most nutrition plans.

CHANGING FOOD HABITS

For some, after abiding by what feels like a lifetime of food preferences and food avoidances, the thought of changing your menu seems daunting. Using spinach as an example, if you didn't learn to like spinach as a child and you didn't find a way to enjoy spinach for the next five-plus decades, you may think there is no hope for spinach in your life. That train left the station a long time ago! This was the case for me, not only with spinach but with many other healthy vegetables. I definitely had a fixed mindset when it came to trying new vegetables!

My diet changed significantly in recent years. About five years ago, after mostly healthy annual physical exam results for many years, I received a letter in the mail from my nurse practitioner summarizing the results of my blood pressure, body mass index, cholesterol levels, blood sugar, and other indicators. In the middle of the letter, she asked if anyone in my family had kidney disease. She went on to say my glomerular filtration rate (GFR) was lower than expected. This was a surprise because there isn't a history of kidney disease in my family, and I didn't have any noticeable symptoms. I felt pretty good! Later, I learned that often there are no symptoms for kidney disease until more damage has been done.

This letter began my quest to learn more about kidney disease and, more importantly, how to prevent future decline. I learned that I am in the "3 percent club," a smaller subset of people who have kidney disease *without* the often associated diabetes (my blood sugar is levels are normal) or high blood pressure (also normal). Still, after retesting, the numbers did not lie, and, despite unknown reasons, I had to accept that I have kidney disease.

To learn more about it, I read whatever I could find on the topic of kidney disease and consulted a dietitian and other providers about kidney-friendly foods and other lifestyle changes. You might say I was motivated to change my food habits by the future threat of kidney dialysis and other physical hardships. I learned meat proteins can increase the acid load to the kidneys and potentially damage kidney cells, and plant-based protein has been found to help preserve function in ailing kidneys (Greger, 2015). Processed meats and meats with additives are also harmful. Eating more fruits and vegetables is also important for kidneys because they help balance the acid load and provide protection from kidney damage (Greger, 2015). Overall, I learned it was important to avoid processed foods whenever possible.

Gradually my GFR has improved, and at the time of this writing, my most recent GFR was within a healthy range (woot-hoot!).

If you have avoided some foods for a while or for a long time, why not give them a second look? Consider ways to gradually add new food items to your existing favorites.

Cravings

Today, we have a homemade poster hanging in our pantry, and this is what it says:

> *Danger: Poison*
> *This is an addictive substance! Worse than cocaine.*
> *This is like alcohol, but without the buzz!*
> *This is the reason we can't stop eating.*
> *It is the culprit behind many chronic diseases.*

The headline on this poster? Sugar.

According to the American Diabetes Association, sugar, especially in the form of sugar-sweetened drinks, has been associated with several serious health problems (Bray, 2014). The article describes a meta-analysis and randomized clinical trials used to evaluate outcomes of beverage and fructose intake. According to the article, 75 percent of all foods and beverages contain added sugars. This bears repeating—75 percent of all foods and beverages contain added sugars! Most of what we put in our mouths has had sugar added to it! The study found lower sugar intake reduced weight gain. Sugar plays a role in obesity, metabolic syndrome, fatty liver disease, and other health problems. Metabolic syndrome is a term for the combined heart and vascular risk factors, including insulin resistance, obesity, atherogenic dyslipidemia, and hypertension—or high blood pressure (Huang, 2009). Atherogenic dyslipidemia is a term for three combined problems: small, dense low-density lipoprotein (LDL) particles; decreased high-density lipoprotein (HDL) particles, and increased triglycerides. All of these health problems are associated with sugar.

Unfortunately, foods we sometimes think of as comfort foods are high in unhealthy starches, fats, and sugars. We enjoy them, and we may even crave them. However, we want to avoid too much of a good thing. So how does one avoid too much sugar, anyway?

BECOME A SUGAR DETECTIVE

It takes more than "just say no to desserts" to avoid added sugars. It requires you to be somewhat of a food detective and a serious food label reader. Added sugars are not only in desserts and many bakery items but also in savory foods like pasta sauce, soup, cereal bars, ketchup, and more. Adding complication are the multiple names for sugar. Here are few: agave nectar, barley malt, barley malt syrup, beet sugar, brown sugar, cane juice, cane juice crystals, cane sugar, caramel, corn syrup, date sugar, demerara sugar, dextrin, dextrose, maltol, maple syrup, molasses, palm sugar, and the list goes on—up to sixty-one names for sugar identified by researchers at the University of California-San Francisco! They promote Sugar Science, a nonprofit organization and source for evidence-based and scientific information about sugar and its impact on health. Some sad facts from Sugar Science:

- Too much added sugar doesn't just make us fat, it can also make us sick.

- Americans consume sixty-six pounds of added sugar on average each year.
- Tobacco conglomerates bought food and drink companies in the early 1960s and developed marketing campaigns to peddle soft drinks.

Unfortunately, added sugar in your diet can give you cravings for, you guessed it, more sugar!

I know all about this because I had to overcome sugar cravings in my quest to eat healthier, though I didn't think of them as "cravings." I just really liked desserts, especially chocolate. As a child, my family drank added sugar in colored drink mixes, and desserts were served with many meals. Of course, healthy foods were always at the table, but there were often sweet snacks in the house. My family especially liked bars—those desserts that have one or more layers of really sweet stuff over a cookie-like crust. Some were fruit-filled, some chocolate-filled, some peanut-y. Some were made with real butter and some with less fattening applesauce or other fruits. Some were crumbly, stuck to the pan, and would not have won a blue ribbon at the county fair. We were not picky.

And no matter how we sliced them, usually twenty-one or twenty-four pieces to a pan, they were devoured by the Hackbarth family—young and old. That's a lot of devouring, especially in a family with five sisters and four brothers. Over the years, we began calculating the size of family events, not by the number of people expected, but by the number of pans of bars we would need. And sometimes there would be lots of pans. Eventually, the dessert table at family gatherings grew to require more card tables.

I'm told some families greet each other with, "It's so nice to see you." Well, with my family it was more like, "Your bars look so nice!"

Some families welcome you at the door and say, "May I take your coat?" With us, it was more like, "May I take your pan?"

Okay, I may be exaggerating a little. Sometimes we did have cookies. You know, those round things? Sometimes we even had cake, for instance, for a birthday. But the bars dominated. They didn't have to be perfect to be appreciated by our clan. They didn't have to look good. They could be too hard, too mushy, a little crumbly, or even have burnt edges. They just had to be there, and we would eat them.

Fast-forward to today, and for all we know about nutrition, you'd think this bar tradition would have been replaced. You'd think that by now we would be salivating over a salad bar, not a dessert bar. The good news is some change has occurred, a definite and noticeable shift. I can't recall the last time our extended family had a nine-pan affair. Today, just one or two pans seem to suffice. But, for some reason, this bar fetish is sticking with us. I think it has something to do with our family name, Hack*BAR*th!

With all confidence, I can say that if I can quit added sugar, so can you. If reducing sugar is something you decide you want to change in your life, it can be done!

Cut Back on Sugar

Mark Hyman, MD, the medical director at Cleveland Clinic's Center for Functional Medicine, has published extensively on sugar and health. Here are a few of his recommendations to help cut back on added sugar:

- Decide to break the sugar habit. Avoid sugar and starch. Quit cold turkey, including sugar substitutes.
- Eat foods with healthy fats to help stave off food cravings.
- Eat your calories. Don't drink them.
- Add protein to every meal, and eat the healthy carbohydrates like non-starchy vegetables.
- Manage your stress. When you are stressed, your cortisol hormone increases, which makes you hungrier.
- Get sufficient sleep.

Some food items can be successfully eliminated by gradually cutting back; however, with added sugars you may struggle if you take this approach. A little added sugar leads to craving for more sugar—it's a vicious cycle. You may find that quitting added sugars cold turkey makes the most sense for you.

Below is an *Amaging™ Affirmation* you may wish to use or adapt to help you eat less sugar.

Figure 10 Stuck on Savory *Amaging*™ Affirmation

Step 1: What do you really want?

I want to eat mostly savory foods (as little added sugar as possible).

Step 2: What is your growth mindset to support this?

I believe I can let go of old eating habits and learn new and better ones.

Step 3: Why do you want it?

I want to maintain a healthy body mass index. I want to be addicted to healthy foods. I want my body to burn more fat, speed up my metabolism, keep my heart healthy, keep my bones strong, and lessen inflammation.

Step 4: What new hat will you wear? Describe what type of person you are willing to become.

I am committed to becoming a careful, mindful food detective who reads food labels and looks for added grams of sugar. I'll become a note taker, recording the number of added sugar grams I consume each day. I'll become mindful and selective, even snobbish at times about what I choose to put in my mouth. I'll become resilient and recognize that when I fall off the wagon, I will need to get right back on to avoid binging on sugar.

Step 5: What are you committed to doing?

I will become a "disciplined foodie" and strive for less than twelve grams of added sugar carbohydrates per day (or another amount recommended by my doctor or health-care provider). I will use healthy spices and healthy vegetables to add flavor to my diet. I will have other food items on hand that do not include sugar, such as sparkling water with lemon rather than a soda. I will avoid my trigger foods that trigger cravings for more sugar. I will weigh myself frequently and record my weight.

Step 6: How will you encourage yourself?

Reinforce your affirmation with inspirational quotes, proverbs, or scripture to build momentum and achieve your goal.

You get fit in the gym, and you lose weight in the kitchen.

—Dr. Timothy Logemann.
(I may exercise often, but I won't drop pounds unless I am consistently mindful of what I put in my mouth.)

The more you eat, the less flavor; the less you eat, the more flavor.

—Chinese Proverb.
(Good nutrition is about quality, not quantity!)

The doctor of the future will give no medication but will interest his patients in the care of the human frame, diet, and in the cause and prevention of disease.

—Thomas A. Edison. (Edison died in 1931; he had great foresight! I can take more personal responsibility for my health by making healthy diet and activity choices.)

> *Do not join those who drink too much wine or gorge themselves on meat, for drunkards and gluttons become poor, and drowsiness clothes them in rags.*
>
> —Proverbs 23:20-22. (God discourages gluttony—overeating.)

Eat Smaller Portions

While sugar may be the challenge for some, for others it's controlling portion sizes, and of course, for some of us, both sugar and portion size may be an issue. The American Diabetes Association recommends portion control as a good way to cut calories and lose extra weight. This way, you don't have to eliminate your favorite foods entirely.

Controlling portion size usually involves three steps:

- seeing how much you eat
- deciding how much to eat
- cutting back on portion size (American Diabetes Society, 2019)

At a restaurant, one way to control portions is to order an appetizer rather than an entrée or to eat half of your order and share your meal. Whenever I can, I try to fill up on the vegetables I like before leaving home. Then, when I'm at the restaurant, I order a protein with a vegetable or salad. If the menu doesn't have a salad or vegetable I particularly enjoy, I know I did not miss out on my required vegetables for that meal because I already ate healthy veggies before leaving the house.

Here are some tips for controlling portion size. These tips were published on MedlinePlus (Wax, Zieve, & Conaway, 2018):

- Do not eat from the bag.
- Serve food on smaller plates.
- For every meal, half of your plate should contain green vegetables.
- Do not eat mindlessly.

Moving from mindless eating (those times when you eat without even thinking about what you are putting in your mouth) to mindful eating can be challenging. It may have taken a lifetime to develop mindless eating habits, so it may take longer than you realize to change them. But, as discussed in the previous paragraphs, it's worth it! A helpful resource on this topic is *The Joy of Half a Cookie*, a book by Jean Kristeller, PhD, and Alisa Bowman. This book describes how to use mindfulness to support weight loss and end food struggles. By being more mindful while eating, you may cultivate a relationship with flavor and nourishment and have more satisfaction with food.

Being in the present moment when eating supports healthy eating habits in many ways. With mindful eating, foods are not allowed or disallowed, but rather you focus on those foods you enjoy more or enjoy less. When mindful, you are conscious of what you truly enjoy—or do not enjoy eating. When you are mindful, you give more attention to your body. You feel relaxed, less obsessive or worried about weight, body image, or cravings. When you are more mindful, you can identify the triggers that lead to overeating. With mindfulness, you can also practice understanding yourself and showing compassion toward yourself. Your food tastes better, and you will likely be surprised to find that you are more satisfied with smaller amounts of food as you become more mindful.

When you eat less, you enjoy your food more. That's important if you decide to work on portion size. By giving more attention to the *quality* of your food, you may be surprised at how much you enjoy eating with less guilt. You may want to use the fill-in-the-blank template in appendix 1 to write an *Amaging™ Affirmation* to support your goal to reduce portion size. You can access a free fillable form for an *Amaging™ Affirmation* at www.amaging.info.

12

Strengthening Our Faith While Growing Old

> "These are the days—the harvest days,
> When life is rich and whole—
> The spirit's golden bounty days.
> Fulfillment of the soul."
> —Helen Lowrie Marshall

God has woven affirmations throughout the Bible. With a little digging into scripture, you may find high-impact verses that speak to you and your current situation. Consider the affirmative language found in a well-known portion of scripture in Psalm 23 (Holy Bible, 2011):

1. The Lord is my shepherd, I lack nothing.
2. He makes me lie down in green pastures, he leads me beside quiet waters,
3. He refreshes my soul. He guides me along the right paths for his name's sake.

> 4 Even though I walk through the darkest valley, I will fear no evil, for you are with me; your rod and your staff, they comfort me.
> 5 You prepare a table before me in the presence of my enemies. You anoint my head with oil; my cup overflows.
> 6 Surely your goodness and love will follow me all the days of my life, and I will dwell in the house of the Lord forever.

This Psalm 23 fits well with my working definition of **an affirmation: the action of declaring something positive and helpful to myself or to other people in a way that will affect positive changes.** The six verses above are positive, can be helpful particularly in times of distress, and help bring about a positive change while also strengthening a person's faith.

Now, use a little imagination and consider how the impact would diminish if Psalm 23 were written with a less affirmative tone, yet had a similar meaning. For example:

> 1 When I am not sure which way to go, the Lord helps me avoid going in the wrong direction, and I don't need to keep wanting for things.
> 2 If I need help, the Lord can guide me to places where I don't have to keep moving or keep looking for food, and places where it isn't too noisy,
> 3 He tries to understand the depths of my emotions and how to make my stressed-out self feel better. He does not point me in bad directions, for his name's sake.
> 4 Even though I am in darker situations, I will try not to be afraid, and I won't need to go looking for God; He offers his rod and His staff to help me if I want to avoid being uncomfortable.
> 5 God makes good things accessible to me, even if my enemies are pretty close by. God can help me avoid being uncomfortable, and I probably will not need more things.
> 6 I'm pretty sure goodness and love are out there for me during my lifetime, and afterward I hope to go to heaven.

Words matter. The second version was my very basic attempt to rewrite in a less positive tone a part of scripture known for its positive, poetic, comforting, and strong affirmations. I have not done these six verses much justice; my version is much less affirming and rather pathetic. But I wanted to illustrate the power of affirmations by contrasting affirmative language with non-affirmative, more neutral language, and even passive word choices.

As a child, I attended a very strict, conservative church in a rural farming community in Wisconsin. In order to learn more about our Christian faith, we studied Bible stories, sang songs, and did related craft projects during Sunday School and later during Confirmation classes on Saturday mornings. "Back in the day" we memorized Bible verses—lots of them!

Memory work was a requirement of being Confirmed. In our religion, being Confirmed, or Confirmation, is a special ceremony when Confirmands (usually teenagers) profess their faith and then can become more involved in the church. After Confirmation, church members can begin to take Communion, the Sacrament of the Lord's Supper with bread and wine representing Christ's body and blood, given for the forgiveness of sins. So, Confirmation was a big deal. Confirmation was not optional. This meant avoiding memory work was not an option.

To prepare for Confirmation, I memorized dozens of Bible verses, which seemed like hundreds or thousands at the time. I did so very reluctantly! Fast-forward four decades after I was confirmed, and as I think back to those painful times spent trying to memorize, I realize I am thankful to have these words placed in my heart. Over time, some of the following Bible verses have been both pain and stress relievers for me:

Psalm 46: God is our refuge and strength, a very present help in trouble.

Romans 8:28: And we know that in all things God works for the good of those who love Him, who have been called according to His purpose.

> *Matthew 6:9-6:12 (The Lord's Prayer) Our Father in heaven, hallowed be your name, your kingdom come, your will be done, on earth as it is in heaven. Give us today our daily bread. And forgive us our debts, as we also have forgiven our debtors. And lead us not into temptation, but deliver us from the evil one.*
>
> *Ephesians 2:4-8: (Grace is undeserved love) For it is by grace you have been saved, through faith—and this not from yourselves, it is the gift of God.*

Notice the affirmative language in the above verses: *refuge, strength, help, deliver, raised us up, gift of God, eternal life,* and others. These comforting verses have stuck with me for more than four decades.

If you are a Christian, you may be not be surprised to learn **your affirmations will be more powerful when you include an inspiring Bible verse as part of your *Amaging*™ *Affirmation*.** This could be in combination with a quote from literature or a stand-alone Bible verse. My Bible has a reference index to look up passages by key word—which is pretty sweet. There are many online Bible resources that allow you to search the Bible quite quickly by typing in a word or few key words, similar to a Google (or other internet) search. I find www.biblegateway.com helpful when writing my personal affirmations.

Using Bible Verses with Affirmations

I follow a Christian blogger, Arabah Joy, who recently shared the story of her ongoing struggle with negativity, and after a Bible study she decided to focus on a specific Bible verse, Philippians 4:8:

> *Finally, brothers and sisters, whatever is true, whatever is noble, whatever is right, whatever is pure, whatever is lovely, whatever is admirable—if anything is excellent or praiseworthy—think about such things.*

She decided to change "Philippians 4:8" from a noun to a verb and apply it to negativity when she noticed pessimism coming out. She would "Philippians 4:8-ercise" situations. If she found herself talking negatively or when the proverbial jar seemed half-empty or less than half, she would ask herself, "Is it true? Noble? Right? Pure? Lovely? Admirable?" This helped her break the habit of negative thinking. She realized some amazing outcomes as well, including more peace of mind and less energy wasted due to destructive thoughts (Playforth, 2019).

Philippians 4:8 would be a high-impact verse to use with step 6 as you write your *Amaging™ Affirmations*. There are many verses you may wish to consider as you create your affirmations. You may choose to read a specific book in the Bible or use a cross-reference function to look up specific Bible verses.

Here are a few examples of scripture you may find helpful:

If your affirmation relates to:	Consider this Bible verse:	
Contentment, Never Giving Up	Philippians 4:12-13	I have learned the secret of being content in any and every situation, whether well fed or hungry, whether living in plenty or in want. I can do all this through him who gives me strength.
Peace of Mind	Matthew 11:28-30	Come to me, all you who are weary and burdened, and I will give you rest. Take my yoke upon you and learn from me, for I am gentle and humble in heart, and you will find rest for your souls. For my yoke is easy and my burden is light.
Joy	Luke 10:20	However, do not rejoice that the spirits submit to you, but rejoice that your names are written in heaven.
Kindness, Compassion, Humility, Gentleness, Patience	Colossians 3:12-13	Therefore, as God's chosen people, holy and dearly loved, clothe yourselves with compassion, kindness, humility, gentleness and patience. Bear with each other and forgive one another if any of you has a grievance against someone. Forgive as the Lord forgave you.

If your affirmation relates to:	Consider this Bible verse:	
Thankfulness, Faithfulness	Psalm 100:4-5	Enter his gates with thanksgiving and his courts with praise; give thanks to him and praise his name. For the Lord is good and his love endures forever; his faithfulness continues through all generations.
Victory, Success	1 Corinthians 15:57 Romans 8:37	But thanks be to God! He gives us the victory through our Lord Jesus Christ. In all these things we are more than conquerors through him who loved us.

Encouragement	Psalm 55:22
	Galatians 6:9
		Cast your cares on the Lord
		   and he will sustain you;
		he will never let
		   the righteous be shaken.
		
		Let us not become weary in doing good, for at the proper time we will reap a harvest if we do not give up.

Help from the Lord	Hebrews 13:6	So we say with confidence, "The Lord is my helper; I will not be afraid. What can mere mortals do to me?"
Reading the Bible More Often	Psalm 119:97	Oh, how I love your law! I meditate on it all day long.
Attending Church More, Praising God	Exodus 15:2	The Lord is my strength and my defense; he has become my salvation. He is my God, and I will praise him, my father's God, and I will exalt him.
Abundant Life	John 10:10 Philippians 4:13	I have come that they may have life, and have it to the full. I can do all things through Christ who strengthens me.
Hope	Jeremiah 29:11 2 Timothy 1:7	For I know the plans I have for you, declares the Lord, plans to prosper you and not to harm you, plans to give you hope and a future. God has not given us a spirit of fear, but of power and love and of sound mind.

A local pastor or other clergy member will be a helpful resource to help you gather more insights from your Bible. You may also want to search the internet for "Bible study" plus any key words relating to your topic, such as healthy eating and Bible study, more exercise and Bible study, meditation and Bible study, or friendship and Bible study. You may be surprised at the number of Bible-based resources available on your chosen topic.

BEGIN WITH THE END IN MIND

A wise hospital administrator and mentor often said to me, "Begin with the end in mind." While planning a meeting, what did I want to accomplish during that hour? While putting a budget together, what was the bottom line I need to work toward? While mapping out a new project, how will the team measure success? While writing a proposal, what was the main takeaway? This simple motto has been useful in my career in many ways and has helped me become more productive. This phrase, "Begin with the end in mind" is also number two in The *7 Habits of Highly Effective People,* a best-selling book about lessons for personal change written by Stephen Covey.

> Picture your future and start planning and working toward it.
> Begin at the end and work backward;
> this makes sense for most goals, including faith-related goals.
> What is the primary ending to keep in mind?

For many of us, from a faith perspective, the ultimate goal relates to what happens after this life and entrance into heaven.

There is a beautiful song made popular by the Afters, and I've left instructions for my family to include this song in my funeral as a reminder of a great celebration and family reunion taking place when I die. God willing, this song will also describe how I lived my life! Each time I hear this song on the radio, I'm reminded that I want to be faithful every day I'm blessed to be on this earth— and then take steps to enjoy the heavenly welcome as described in this song. I try to begin each day with "Well Done" in mind.

> *What will it be like when You call my name*
> *And that moment when I see You face-to-face?*
> *I'm waiting my whole life to hear You say*
> *Well done, well done*
> *My good and faithful one*
> *Welcome to the place where you belong…* (Ingram, 2018)
>
> —"Well Done" by the Afters

Amaging™ and Vulnerable

A wonderful geriatrician I had the honor of consulting with earlier in my career had a way of pulling a key adjective into his vocabulary frequently when talking about older adults who were sick or injured. This adjective was "vulnerable." He seldom referred to elders without saying, "vulnerable elder(s)." He used the term "vulnerable" in a good way to remind his colleagues, team members, and others that their work was important. The patients and families he and his care team supported needed clinicians willing to support challenges of a highly vulnerable patient population.

As our years increase, often life's challenges increase as well. While we strive to be more *amaging*™, it's likely we will also become more vulnerable in the face of challenges as we age. Here are a few examples of common vulnerabilities for older adults:

- less physical ability to do activities we enjoy
- less energy to take on some activities

- more ongoing or chronic health conditions that may require new lifestyle habits and new coping skills
- fewer friends (as discussed in chapter 9) due to changes in geography, housing, death, and other reasons
- more frustration when mobility or independence declines
- aggravating negative stereotypes and attitudes about aging
- more health-care expenses
- more financial worries and constraints due to a fixed income

If you were to pause here and reflect on the variety of trials in your life, or your parents' or grandparents' lives as they grew older, it's likely you will agree that older adults face many obstacles. Elders are vulnerable.

A strong prayer life can help support a growth mindset during this part of life's journey. As you reflect on your challenges relating to growing older, consider how you might pray for the grace to surrender them to God.

Here's an example of a prayer I wrote to help me have a better frame of mind while growing older:

> *Dear God. I do not know what the future holds. As I picture an older version of myself, with more struggles, pain, and difficult experiences, I am sometimes anxious about this. I pray that I will avoid focusing on negative thoughts like self-pity, frustration, or anger. Rather, I pray that I will grow closer to you, and I will put daily challenges in Your hands. I pray my relationship with You will become stronger and more intimate each day as I grow older—until I take my final breath, and my life is truly in Your hands.*

As you think about becoming more physically vulnerable and the challenges ahead, what makes you most anxious? Take it to the Lord in prayer. Prayer helps offset, "Thinking with the Enemy," as discussed in chapter 7.

A stronger prayer life can help support many of the topics in this book. Consider how you might use prayer to do all or some of the following:

- build new, healthier habits
- be more self-compassionate
- be more positive about growing older
- be a better friend
- make new friends
- move more, be more active
- be more resourceful
- eat healthier
- pray more

Prayers can also be used in combination with the *Amaging*™ *Affirmation* framework. In the *Amaging*™ *Framework's* step 6, "Encourage Yourself," you may wish to replace this step with something like, "How can I take this to the Lord in prayer?" Supercharge your encouragement by adding a prayer to step 6. Another option might be to add a step 7 and write yourself a simple prayer to support your *Amaging*™ *Affirmation*. If praying is something new to you, or if you are experienced at prayer but would like more consistency, you may wish to use or adapt the following *Amaging*™ *Affirmation* to improve your prayer life.

FIGURE 11 *AMAGING*™ *AFFIRMATION* TO PRAY MORE

Step 1: What do you really want?

I want a two-way conversation with God and a stronger relationship with Him. I want to shift my mindset, viewing prayer as a privilege, not an obligation. I want to pray boldly not because I understand *how* God makes things work but because I am convinced God loves me, hears me, and answers my prayers.

Step 2: What is your growth mindset to support this?

I believe prayer works. I can learn to pray better and more consistently.

Step 3: Why do you want it?

I want God's will for my life. I want a stronger prayer life because without prayer I may become weaker and more easily lured into negativity and other sins. I want to seek and give forgiveness. I want to give thanks. I want to follow God's commands, as he tells us to pray: "Continue earnestly in prayer, being vigilant in it with thanksgiving" (Colossians 4:2).

Step 4: What new hat will you wear? Describe what type of person you are willing to become.

I will become the type of person who accepts "no" for an answer, and I trust that the answer to my prayers cannot always be a "yes." I want to be the type of person who embraces humility, recognizing that only God is all-knowing. I want to be the type of person who can give up control, trusting that God knows both the future and the past, and what is good or bad for me.

Step 5: What are you committed to doing? Be specific.

I will proactively improve my routine of praying. I will maintain a prayer list of prayers to say on a rotation (for instance, prayers for my husband, family, co-workers, etc.) and I will maintain a list of special prayers for special needs. I will find an online tool with a simple checklist function to help manage both of my prayer lists. I will look for prayer triggers, like when I hear a rescue siren going by, when I learn someone is in trouble or hurting, when there are natural disasters, when I'm stuck in uncertainty, distress, or simply annoyed.

Step 6: How will you encourage yourself?

Encourage yourself! Reinforce your affirmation with one or more inspirational quotes, proverbs, *or* scripture to build momentum and achieve your goal. Don't skimp on this step.

> *Prayer is simply talking to God like a friend and should be the easiest thing we do each day.*
>
> —Joyce Meyer

> *Do not be anxious about anything, but in everything, by prayer and petition, with thanksgiving, present your requests to God.*
>
> —Philippians 4:6

> *Don't forget to pray today, because God did not forget to wake you up this morning.*
>
> —Unknown

> *Ask and it will be given to you; seek and you will find; knock and the door will be opened to you. For everyone who asks receives; he who seeks finds; and to him who knocks, the door will be opened.*
>
> —Matthew 7:7-8.

> *Faith in God includes faith in His timing.*
>
> —Neal A. Maxwell

> *Is prayer your steering wheel or your spare tire?*
>
> —Corrie ten Boom

> *To be a Christian without prayer is no more possible than to be alive without breathing.*
>
> —Martin Luther

Age Bias and Affirmations: Replace Fear with Faith

In his book, *The Hope Quotient*, Ray Johnston talks about looking beyond our cognitive intelligence and our emotional intelligence to also explore the next level of intelligence, which he describes as our hope quotient (Johnston, 2014). In his career, Johnston has analyzed factors that help people become more hopeful, and, by moving in this more hopeful direction, he asserts that anything is possible.

Here are some ways additional hopefulness, even a 10 percent improvement in one's "hope quotient" can make a difference:

- start on a path to getting in shape physically
- break bad habits
- find new energy to support children
- feel inspired to apply for a new job or return to school
- connect more with God for spiritual health (Johnston, 2014)

Sometimes, as more years are lived, our spirit of hopefulness declines. Without realizing it, we may have acquired a fear of growing old. As described in chapter 4, age bias chips away at our positive attitudes about growing older. Unconscious age bias can be present when we are unaware, and more optimism about aging has been studied and shown to add 7.5 years of life. In his discussion about the hope quotient, Johnston illustrates how faith can help overcome fear.

Are there ways older adults might lean on their faith to help tackle the fear of aging, which is reinforced by age bias in our culture? Some of the destructive elements of age bias are discussed in chapter 4, and they include the following:

> F—Focusing on the problem (the physical decline of aging, the loss of career relationships and rewards, financial challenges, and other inabilities associated with growing older).

E—Expectation of defeat (with each new day and each new year, things feel like they are getting worse).

A—Attitude of self-protection (avoiding obstacles that seem too great for an older adult, rather than developing a plan with small or big steps to overcome).

R—Running from the problem (giving in, losing hope, feeling defeated).

Now, consider how faith might be used to move past the fear of aging. Do any of these fearful elements ring true for you? By focusing more on God and less on your problems, anticipating God's help, improving your prayer life, believing you have a Savior, and recognizing other elements of faith, your faith can help you offset the fears associated with aging.

The *Amaging*™ *Affirmations* framework in this book can be used to help you become more hopeful while growing older, at a time when the culture of age bias may diminish our hope. In figure 11, I wrote an affirmation to help enhance my prayer life. You may want to tweak or adapt this to help you strengthen your faith and overcome your personal fears and struggles. In chapter 14, I'll venture more deeply into using *Amaging*™ *Affirmations* to help overcome fears.

13

The Pain Is Real and So Is the Fatigue

My dear friend, I don't want to ignore what may be the so-called elephant in the room when talking about growing older. Writing about positive attitudes toward aging, mindset, using affirmations, and staying encouraged may give the impression that pain, fatigue, and other difficult symptoms are not significant. Of course, this is not the case. Older adults often have ongoing and complex health conditions accompanied by symptoms of pain, fatigue, shortness of breath, chills, fever, lightheadedness, nausea, heavy thirst, weakness, and other physical symptoms. These symptoms are real, and they can be incredibly uncomfortable, sometimes unbearable.

These symptoms, combined with a loss of physical function, can lead to less independence—which means more dependence on other people for things like driving, making meals, getting dressed in the morning, showering, going shopping, and just moving around. As one becomes less independent, the struggles of growing older become worse. While questioning older adults for this book, one man in his sixties shared:

> *It's frustrating to deal with the reality that how I am feeling or my health status on a daily basis is the major factor in deciding the level of activity I can engage in on any given day.*

In this book, I've shared a few stories about people who have faced painful and difficult obstacles. Among other health problems, my friend Ginny required assisted living support and experienced painful osteoporosis. Hal Elrod, an author who I consider my mentor, has written and shared in his podcasts many stories about his rehabilitation and painful recovery after a vehicle crash, which left him with multiple injuries, including the loss of short-term memory from a traumatic brain injury. Later, Elrod survived excruciating pain and fatigue from cancer treatments. I also shared the story of Sarah, an incarcerated Christian who wants to leave a legacy of someone whose love for Jesus turned an angry heart into a loving one—and restored her soul. No doubt, Sarah suffers from mental anguish, loneliness, and the daily stressors of prison life. Scott Rigsby, described in chapter 6, described his pain as his "new normal." He was seriously injured in a vehicle crash, leaving him with one leg amputated and the other leg badly injured. Rigsby suffered a traumatic brain injury, had multiple surgeries, panic attacks, constant pain, depression, and later a sleeping disorder. (I counted my own blessings many times while reading his autobiography.) Jeff Krause, my former choir director, experienced the pain associated with serious illnesses—an organ transplant, a heart condition, and cancer.

While doing research for this book, I interviewed a friend from elementary and high school whom I had not spoken with for any length of time in years. She was kind enough to sit down with me and share more about some of her age-related issues. Very early in the conversation, I learned she is definitely an *amaging*™ person! She said she does not want to follow that fragile path of aging. She is active, with a full-time job, enjoys gardening, house renovating, and has many family commitments. And, in her spare time, she trains to run marathons! Later in life she discovered her joy in running. Still, when it comes to growing older, her greatest problem is fatigue, which is an overall feeling of tiredness or lack of energy. Despite her very active lifestyle, she struggles with fatigue. The good news is that she is seeking medical help to find the cause and a treatment that works.

Another older adult I talked to while researching this book told me that one of his biggest aging challenges is getting good sleep. Now in his seventies, he said his quality of sleep has declined due to restless leg syndrome:

> *I feel that a poor night's sleep affects me in many other negative ways, including next-day fatigue, being less mentally sharp the next day, and overall health.*

He is receiving treatment for this condition and also trying self-massage on his legs, practicing tai chi, and using plant-based supplements.

In each of these examples, a growth mindset, a willingness to "wear a new hat," grow friendships, or take steps toward new lifestyle habits, has helped these amazing people live with pain, fatigue, and other symptoms. My prayer is that there will be words, phrases, and sections of this book that speak to people struggling with difficult symptoms associated with growing older.

While the concepts in this book do not replace medical care, they can support healing and complement your health-care provider's recommendations. If difficult symptoms make your life more problematic, you may find the topics throughout this book, particularly one of the following chapters, helpful:

- Friendships, chapter 9, page 91
- Fitness, chapter 10, page 105
- Food, chapter 11, page 117
- Faith, chapter 12, page 129

14

Practice Makes Better

"Success is the sum of small efforts, repeated day in and day out."
—Robert Collier, author of The Secret of the Ages

"Perfection paralysis" is a term describing a fear that becomes so great it stops us from taking action.

You may experience perfection paralysis if you have decided to wait for ideal conditions before starting or continuing a project. This fear may be a fear of failure, a fear of being judged, a fear of losing credibility, or another type of fear. I experienced this when writing this book, putting off writing for even months at a time, convincing myself there would be better days and blocks of "quiet time" ahead to focus on my book project. While researching how to write a nonfiction book, I learned that the average new writer writes for just thirty minutes to one hour per day. The average new writer doesn't wait for the perfect day, week, month, or year, but rather builds a daily habit.

What fears slowed my writing? A lot of them! Here are a few:

- fear of not doing enough research on the key points in the book

- fear of not being able to manage my day job well enough to write after hours
- fear of making a mistake and misstating or misquoting something important
- fear of failure and writing a book that isn't read

The list goes on! I was "thinking with the enemy" too often. For me, I find I need to push myself to start something and course correct later. Get started. Practice, and trust the practice will help improve the task at hand.

When the COVID-19 pandemic arrived, many sewing enthusiasts found themselves frantically sewing masks for themselves, loved ones, local hospitals, and for others. While I enjoy sewing, I found perfection paralysis set in rather quickly. First, I hunted for the ideal mask pattern that was as close to the fitted N95 mask as possible. But I also needed it to be rather easy to sew. One of the best patterns I found seemed to qualify, but there were no written instructions. An art teacher created a forty-five-minute step-by-step video, and it was intended for those who don't normally sew. After making one rather tedious and surprisingly fitted mock-up, I decided I had to look for a new pattern, because I wanted something with simpler instructions to reference—not a long video tutorial.

Once I finally settled on a pattern, I began the drawn-out task of researching the ideal fabric to use for droplet precautions. Or should it be a combination of fabrics with a removable filtering layer? Interestingly, I found much was written on this topic—adding to my perfection paralysis! In the end, I settled on two layers of high-quality quilting fabric. Fortunately, I had a small stash of fabric that qualified in my sewing closet. Then I began the color selection, followed by the thread selection. At one point, I wondered if the pandemic storm would end before I finished sewing my first mask (not that that would be a bad thing)! In the end, I made a handful of masks for me and my husband. My sister didn't have the same decision-making dilemma I did. She found her pattern right away, dug into her fabric collection, and started sewing.

With your planning, I suggest you act more like my sister and less like me; don't let perfection paralysis stop you from moving forward.

Knowledge Is a Great Start, yet Not Enough to Change Behavior

In my career, I had the good fortune to connect with and even work for the Wisconsin Institute for Healthy Aging (WIHA). This is a nonprofit organization with a goal to become a one-stop shop for scientifically proven self-management education programs. One of WIHA's flagship programs is Stepping On, a researched falls-prevention program to help older adults walk more confidently. I have a lot of knowledge of this program, the risk factors for falls, and the strategies recommended to prevent a fall. Some of these strategies include building and maintaining strength and balance, wearing proper footwear, understanding medications, avoiding alcohol, modifying the home environment, using care when walking on ice and snow, and other strategies.

I worked with a team to help bring this program to older adults in central and northern Wisconsin, and later I had the privilege of helping disseminate Stepping On to health systems and other organizations throughout North America. I frequently talked with injury-prevention specialists, education coordinators for aging programs, and other professionals across the United States who care deeply about falls prevention and want to help older adults avoid falling. I learned from and worked closely with WIHA experts and clinicians to understand the program and its benefits. I knew falls prevention.

Unfortunately, all of this knowledge did not translate when it came to my own behavior. If anything, I wonder if my knowledge of falls prevention led me to think I *knew* enough to avoid falls and therefore I didn't need to *apply and practice* what I'd learned. My mindset changed after a bad fall.

On the Saturday before Christmas in 2019, I enjoyed a Christmas party before watching a Badger basketball game at the University of Wisconsin-Madison with my family. After the basketball game, we watched a Badger NCAA Championship Volleyball match on television together. It was such a fun day to hang out with my husband and our adult children. Afterward, we walked to a restaurant for dinner, a few blocks from my daughter's apartment. While leaving, I was not paying attention and slipped on a small stretch of ice as I hurried to cross the street. My arms started flailing as I attempted to catch myself, and I hit the pavement hard on my right extended arm. I couldn't move and only felt pain on my right side.

My daughter said that I told her right away that I thought my arm was broken. I don't remember saying this. I only remember the pain and a creepy feeling, watching and trying to feel my right hand as I lost all sensation in each finger, one by one, until my hand just flopped down and couldn't hold itself up. The creepiness of my now flopping hand was matched by the pain in my right arm and shoulder. Mostly, I just closed my eyes and cried. At the hospital, I couldn't tell you much about the nurses or exam room because I kept my eyes shut most of the time. My youngest daughter figured out how to slowly take my jacket off, and a very patient emergency room team cut my sweater, T-shirt, and bra off of me and somehow got me into a gown. After a lot of pain medications (bless the physician assistant who prescribed them) and X-rays, I learned that my right shoulder was dislocated and my right humerus bone was broken near the shoulder. The physician assistant did a quick and impressive manipulation to put the shoulder back into place, and I was sent home with a pain medication prescription and instructions to see an orthopedic surgeon.

At the time of this book's publication, I exercise to build strength, and I'm optimistic I will gain strength and stay active for the long haul, so I can continue to play golf, ride a bike, swim laps, play pickleball, straighten my hair, and possibly sweep a floor again. No rush for the latter!

I'm sharing this falls story not for a sympathy vote but rather to illustrate how **knowledge did not translate into a behavior change** for me. It was a start, yet not enough. I knew the risk factors for falls, yet I fell any way. After reflection, I later counted two factors that I ignored and most likely led to my fall: (1) I did not "walk like a penguin" with a wider stance and short, slow steps on a slippery stretch, but rather I tried to hustle across the street; and (2) I was wearing improper footwear. My older daughter checked out my shoes in the emergency room, and she pointed out they were quite smooth with little traction. We threw them in the garbage along with the clothing they'd cut from my body. I definitely knew better than to wear those shoes in the winter.

While doing research for this book, I asked people about their struggles with growing older. One woman in her mid-sixties said our generation is more fortunate because more is known and shared today about prevention to help us as we age.

> *I don't think doctors used to tell you as much as they do nowadays, and dietitians play such an important role. I don't believe people knew they could go blind from diabetes, or suffer from smoking, and the risks of obesity. In [her community] we do beginner yoga and easy exercise that can then advance to more complex exercise. They also bring in experts to cook and discuss good habits.*

There is no shortage of wellness and prevention information available today. We are inundated with messages to expand our healthy aging knowledge base.

If you have read this far into this book, you have gained some knowledge about growing old in a healthy way. Or, at least that is my hope. Please don't do what I did with the fall prevention knowledge.

Take some slow and careful steps to *apply* what you have learned in this book to set achievable goals, write your own *Amaging™ Affirmations*, use your *Amaging™ Affirmations* to help modify your behaviors. **Practice makes better.**

Start Small and Gain Momentum

Joe Piscatella, mentioned earlier in this book, shared his personal struggle to adopt heart-healthy habits. He said, at first he thought he had to do everything to the extreme right away—run an entire marathon, become a vegetarian, meditate every day—all within two weeks. He set unrealistic goals, and as you can imagine, he wasn't successful.

He wrote, "Then, I realized that a different strategy might be more effective: small actions, repeated daily." He started eating more vegetables at dinnertime. He worked on this until it was a daily dinner habit. Then he worked on eating more fish, and later he tackled portion control. He started with something small and built little successes upon little successes. These little successes became the foundation for his new and healthier life (Piscatella, 2010).

In an online community I follow, another follower said she struggled with setting new intentions, only to give up after a day or two. She asked how others are able to stick to new goals and habits. Great question! A number of people in this online community said they struggled in the same way, and others offered helpful ideas. One member of this community suggested starting with a small habit and making it a daily habit. The reader suggested that she begin by doing something easy like making her bed every day because this small success will provide the confidence to stick to other goals. Another reader suggested taking it slow; don't start with too many new habits at one time. Just change one thing to begin, and then slowly add more and more.

Here is a summary of the many ideas shared, not by experts but by people who are working on reaching goals and practicing new habits:

- **Write** your new habit on a sticky note and keep it on your desk or right in front of you, so you can check off your progress.
- **Plan** your day (see chapter 6).
- You need to **up your belief**. If you don't think the things you want are possible, it will be easy to quit.

- Make this part of your **affirmations**. Some examples were offered: "I will focus on sticking to things. I will follow through and achieve the goals I set for myself…" Or perhaps, "I will keep my commitments to myself and press on in the face of setbacks." Consider adding, "I am worthy" to your affirmations.
- **Change your mindset.** If you tell yourself you suck at sticking to things, your brain may make it a reality.
- Watch the *Five Second Rule* on YouTube by Mel Robins. She suggests using a mantra. One example might be, "It's gonna suck. Do it anyway!"
- Sometimes you just need to **show up**.
- If you really want something, you'll **figure out a way**. If you don't really want it, you'll find an excuse.
- Find an **accountability partner** to hold you to your new goal or action plan. Or find a mentor.
- Consider a **gratitude journal** to shift your mindset when you are feeling down.
- **Don't give up**. Every time you restart, it's a little better than the last.
- **You are capable** of anything. Stop believing the lie that you are not.

Before moving off the topic of practicing and taking intentional steps to become a better person, I want to mention a key concept published by Dr. Brené Brown in her book *Daring Greatly*. Dr. Brown is a researcher on shame, vulnerability, and fear, and she has interviewed and collected stories from thousands of people about their life experiences, behaviors, and emotions. Through her work, Dr. Brown identified some strategies people have used to deal with difficult events and emotions without closing their hearts, a concept she calls, "Wholehearted Living." She and a team of researchers identified a set of "Guideposts for Wholehearted Living." These guideposts cover topics like authenticity, self-compassion, gratitude, creativity, and play and rest, to name a few. Interestingly, each guidepost begins with the word "cultivating," which means to acquire or develop a quality, sentiment, or skill (Dictionary.com, 2019).

Wholehearted people are acquiring, cultivating, and practicing their skills, and at the same time they are working to reduce or eliminate the things in their lives they believe are important to let go.

Below is an *Amaging™ Affirmation* you may want to use to help you practice new habits.

Figure 12 New Habit Affirmation

Step 1: What do you really want?

I want to practice new habits more consistently without getting stuck by perfectionism.

Step 2: What is your growth mindset to support this?

Practice makes better. If I want to be successful, I will probably make some mistakes along the way; I can learn from my mistakes without getting stalled by them.

Step 3: Why do you want it?

This new habit will give me fulfillment because _____.
It will help me do _____, and I will feel _____.

Step 4: What new hat will you wear? Describe what type of person you are willing to become.

A doer. Reading, planning, and reflection are good, but action is better, and even baby steps can move me closer to a consistent habit. A "fruit picker," someone who can grab "low-hanging fruit" and discover quick, small wins to help move my new habit forward and boost my enthusiasm. A problem solver, someone who finds ways to overcome barriers and get back on track. My biggest fan, someone who cheers me on, practices self-compassion, avoids thinking with the enemy (see chapter 7).

Step 5: What are you committed to doing? Be specific.

Complete an *Amaging™ Affirmation & Action Plan* (See appendix 1) to support my new habit. Track my progress on a routine basis, such as weekly or daily, with an eye toward consistency. Use automatic tracking, like a fitness tracker or pedometer, when feasible. When appropriate, use a manual habit tracker (a simple chart or a fancy planner, either will work) when automation is not feasible.

Step 6: How will you encourage yourself?

Reinforce your affirmation with one or more inspirational quotes, proverbs, or scripture to build momentum and achieve your goal. Don't skimp on this step.

> *If you want to step into your greatness, you need to recognize that life will get harder before it gets easier.*
>
> *—Allison Liddle*

> *With this in mind, we constantly pray for you, that our God may make you worthy of his calling, and that by his power he may bring to fruition your every desire for goodness and your every deed prompted by faith. We pray this so that the name of our Lord Jesus may be glorified in you, and you in him, according to the grace of our God and the Lord Jesus Christ.*
>
> *—2 Thesolonians:11-12*

> *We can choose to be perfect and admired or to be real and loved.*
>
> *—Glennon Doyle*

At its root, perfectionism isn't really about a deep love of being meticulous. It's about fear. Fear of making a mistake. Fear of disappointing others. Fear of failure. Fear of success.

—*Michael Law*

15

End on a High Note

> "Live each and every day as if it were your
> last—because one day you'll be right."
> —Bob Moawad

In her book, *How to Have a Good Day*, referenced in the earlier section on brain power, author Caroline Webb explains how to apply science to daily living in order to have good days. Webb lists numerous scientific findings related to perceptions of good days, including the "peak-end effect" which shows how people typically evaluate their happiness levels. When people remember how their day was, they tend to think about an average of the most intense moments (the peak) and then how it ended (the end).

An important implication from the peak-end effect research is to be more intentional, and even systematic, about how we end something—a task, a meeting, a day, a project, even a lifetime—on a high note.

Webb gives some helpful suggestions for ways to end things on a high note:

- At the end of each day, write down or think about **three good things** that happened that day. This is a helpful way to change how you will remember the day for the better.
- When ending a conversation, **recap the most upbeat part** of the conversation. Bring back the positive. Something like, "It was great to hear about…"
- If you are leading a group, before you part ways **ask people what went well** during your time together (Webb, 2016).

While it's always nice to have those peak positive moments, it turns out the *ending* has disproportionately greater impact on overall perceptions of positive experiences. This may be why entertainers put so much energy into grand finales and why grand finales often are pretty grand. As an older adult, what are all the ways you can be more intentional about this part of life's journey? Perhaps take advantage of the peak-end concept to improve your overall perception of a positive life!

People who know me well know that I love, love, love to sing. I sing at home, in the car, while walking—whenever I can. Sometimes I just hum. I'm not very apologetic to the people I annoy with this obsession, either. When I can, I sing with my church choir. Since high school, I have sung second soprano. This means I sing higher notes than altos and usually lower notes than first sopranos. It's a middle part, often sung by female voices. Depending on how the composer puts the choral parts together, this also means I get to sing harmony—as typically first sopranos sing melody. Sometimes when the notes get higher than I would like, I roll my eyes and think, "That's too high for a second soprano" or "That's too high for me."

Sometimes I adopt an ageist attitude and think, "I'm too old to sing that high." Over time, I lost some of my vocal range, and my highest note dropped down to an F in the octave above middle C. I resigned myself to the belief that God made first sopranos to sing higher notes and that second sopranos shouldn't be expected to sing them. I believed that I didn't need to work on my vocal range because I probably couldn't get those high notes back, anyway.

This changed when I had the good fortune to sing with an interfaith Christian community in a performance of *Lamb of God* by Rob Gardner. To say the composer wrote very beautiful music is an understatement. For me the complex rhythm and harmony made the music super hard to learn, and much to my dismay, it included very high notes for both first and *second* sopranos. Because the music was so challenging, I practiced often. Mostly, I practiced in my car on the way to and from work or on road trips. At first, I would lip-synch when I couldn't hit the higher notes.

One day at rehearsal, as I sat quietly and listened to all of the parts sung together, I realized that if I kept lip-synching the notes, there might not be enough second soprano sound in the choir to bring out the composer's really pretty harmony. I decided to try to hit the higher notes and make the attempt to sing them during rehearsal. I decided to think that I could try it. No more lip-synching the high notes! Over time—because I was practicing, practicing, practicing—and when my vocal cords were warmed up, I noticed some of the higher notes gradually came back. By the time of the performance, I was able to sing a G-sharp without it sounding too terrible. My range had increased a full note and a half. This may sound trivial, but I surprised myself. In my middle fifties, I was able to hit a note I hadn't been able to hit in decades, probably not since high school.

I wrote this *Amaging™ Affirmation* for older adults who want to set and achieve a challenging goal.

Feel free to adapt this to make it your own. Many of the strategies in this affirmation come from the book, *The Miracle Equation* (Elrod H. , 2019).

Figure 13 *Amaging*™ Affirmation on Achieving Goals

Step 1: What do you really want?

I want to reflect on and consider the possibilities that lie ahead. I want to set goals that matter to me and then consistently execute them.

Step 2: What is your growth mindset to support this?

I believe I can do this. I have unwavering faith in the real possibilities ahead of me to help me achieve this goal. *Describe your guiding compass to help you get to where you want to be with your goal(s):*
_____.

Step 3: Why do you want it?

I want to tap the potential I know I have. I have accomplished much throughout my life, and I want to build on what I have learned and built up along the way. I want to overcome some self-imposed limits I may have had in the past and win this goal. I want to reach higher because _____.

Step 4: What new hat will you wear? Describe what type of person you are willing to become.

A processor—someone who figures out what steps I need to take to achieve my goal. An inner peacekeeper—someone who maintains peace of mind and stays focused on the process, avoiding any frustration or anxiety that may come with obsessing about the end goal. A scheduler—someone who updates and closely follows a calendar to make time for the process I set up to achieve this goal. A team player who is open to finding an accountability partner(s), asking someone else to hold me responsible, not attempting to "fly solo" with this goal. An adapter—someone who monitors my processes and makes changes along the way.

Step 5: What are you committed to doing? Be specific.

I am willing to put in extraordinary effort to achieve the goal(s). I will find ways to make this "extraordinary effort" as ordinary as possible by adopting simple processes. Then, I will consistently work these processes, scheduling and monitoring my way to success. Here are some specific steps I will take to win this goal:

_____.

Step 6: How will you encourage yourself?

Reinforce your affirmation with one or more inspirational quotes, proverbs, or scripture to build momentum and achieve your goal. Don't skimp on this step.

> *When you live with unwavering faith and put forth extraordinary effort, you are a miracle maven...From the beginning of time, otherwise ordinary people have catapulted themselves beyond the limits of what was thought to be possible. They, too, have had to overcome the same types of fears and insecurities that chain us all.*
>
> —Hal Elrod

> *May He give you the desire of your heart and make all your plans succeed.*
>
> —Psalm 20:4

> *Most impossible goals can be met simply by breaking them down into bite-size chunks, writing them down, believing them and going full speed ahead as if they were routine.*
>
> —Don Lancaster

After hitting the G-sharp for the *Lamb of God* performance, I couldn't help but wonder what other lower notes I was settling for of late. Do I accept the status quo without challenging myself to try a little harder? Practice more? Warm myself up for higher aspirations?

> As an older adult, this part of life's journey
> can be a time to either settle or set.
> Settle for less than your potential or
> set goals to achieve more and amazing—*amaging*™—things.

Can you use this time in your life to set an example for those around you? Perhaps grandchildren who look up to you? Your adult children experiencing stress or struggling with careers, parenting, or work responsibilities? Another volunteer at a local nonprofit? Friends at your church? Others whom God has placed in your life? What aspects of your life might a growth mindset help improve? Your faith? Friendships? Fitness levels?

Set goals. Use the page found in appendix 1 to simplify your planning. Use *Amaging*™ *Affirmations* to help you reach and surpass your goals. Develop new and healthy habits. Continue to learn and practice.

Then look back and enjoy peace of mind, knowing you did all you could to end this life on a high note.

LET'S STAY CONNECTED

Thank you for reading *Amaging*™ **Growing Old On Purpose**.

I invite you to visit www.amaging.info for updates and free resources.

Your feedback regarding this book will be welcomed and appreciated.

—Margie Hackbarth, Author

APPENDIX 1

Amaging™ Affirmation and Action Plan

Step 1: What do you really want? **Step 2**: What is your growth mindset to support this?	

Step 3: Why do you want it?
 	
 Step 4: What new hat will you wear? Describe what type of person you are willing to become.
	Step 5: What are you committed to doing? Be specific.
	
	 Action Plan:
	 Key milestone: By when:
	    Task A
	    Task B
	    Task C
	
	 Key milestone: By when:
	    Task A
	    Task B
	    Task C

Step 6: How will you encourage yourself? Reinforce your affirmation with inspirational quotes, proverbs, or scripture to build momentum and achieve your goal. Don't skimp on this step! Add a new page, if needed.	**Optional–Mini vision board:** Draw or paste an image demonstrating success with a step, milestone, or task relating to this goal.
© 2021 Amaging LLC. All rights reserved. Permission is granted to use this form for your individual use. Group use, sharing this form on social media, or other ways are not permitted.	You may access a free fillable form for an *Amaging™ Affirmation* at www.amaging.info.

Works Cited

Agus, D. M. (2014). *A Short Guide to a Long Life.* New York: Simon & Schuster.

Alidina, S. (2015). *The Mindful Way Through Stress: The Proven Eight-week Path to Health, Happiness, and Well-Being.* New York: The Guilford Press.

American Diabetes Society. (2019). Food and Portion Size. Arlington, VA.

Andrews, E. (2018, August 22). *Seven Late Life Success Stories.* Retrieved May 2019, from History: https://www.history.com/news/7-late-life-success-stories

Applewhite, A. (2016). *This Chair Rocks: A Manesfesto Against Ageism.* Networked Books.

Atighehchi, A., Banayan, A., & Ahdoot, M. (2019). *Morning Sidekick Journal.* Every Damn Day, LLC.

Baker, B. (2017). Commissioner of Health, City of Milwaukee Health Department. *American College of Healthcare Executives.* Elkhart Lake, WI.

Bliezner, R. (2014). The Worth of Friendship: Can Friends Keep us Happy and Healthy? *Generations, 38*(1), 24-29.

Bray, G. A. (2014). Dietary Sugar and Body Weight: Have We Reached a Crisis in the Epidemic of Obesity and Diabetes? *37(4): 950-956*(April 2014). Retrieved from https://doi.org/10.2337/dc13-2085

Brody, J. (2017, April 17). The Cost of Not Taking Your Medicine. *The New York Times*, p. D7.

Brown, B. (2012). *Daring Greatly: How the Courage to Be Vulnerable Transforms the Way We Live, Love, Parent and Lead.* New York: Avery.

Buettner, D. (2012). *The Blue Zones: Nine Lessons for Living Longer.* Washington, D.C.: National Geographic Society.

Canfield, J. (2017). *"Think This, Not That: Your Guide to Everyday Positive Thinking".* Self-Esteem Seminars, LP, JackCanfield.com.

Canfield, J. (2017, February 9). *YouTube.* Retrieved from Stop Using These Affirmations Right Now: https://www.youtube.com/watch?v=LO5FXjc1QdY

Carter, J. (1998). *The Virtues of Aging.* New York: Random House.

Clear, J. (2018). *Atomic Habits: Tiny Changes, Remarkable Results.* New York: Avery.

Cohen, G., & Sherman, D. (2014). The Psychology of Change: Self-Affirmation and Social Psychological Intervention. *Annual Review of Psychology, 65*(https://doi.org/10.1146/annurev-psych-010213-115137), 333-371.

Crocker, J. N. (2008). Why does writing about important values reduce defensiveness? Self-affirmation and the role of positive other-directed feelings. *Psychological Science*(19), 740-747.

Csikszentmihalyi, M. (2008). *Flow: The Psychology of Optimal Experience.* New York: Harper Perennial Modern Classics.

Dictionary.com. (2019, October 7). Random House Unabridged Dictionary.

Duckworth, A. (2018). *Grit: The Power of Passion and Perseverance.* New York City: Scribner.

Dweck, C. S. (2007). *Mindset: The New Psychology of Success.* New York: Ballantine Books.

Ehrenfeld, T. (2017, June 19). To Age Well, You Need Friends. *Psychology Today.*

Elrod, H. (2012). *The Miracle Morning.* Hal Elrod International, Inc.

Elrod, H. (2019). *The Miracle Equation: : The Two Decisions That Move Your Biggest Goals from Possible, to Probable, to Inevitable.* New York: Harmony.

Epton, T. H. (2008). Self-affirmation promotes health behavior change. *Health Psychology, 27,* 746-752.

Falk, E. B. (2015). Self-affirmation alters the brain's response to health messages and subsequent behavior change. *Proceedings of the National Academy of Sciences of the United States of America.* Retrieved 2017, from https://www.ncbi.nlm.nih.gov/pmc/articles/PMC4343089/

Ferrari, N. (2017, March 1). *50 Ways to Live a Longer, Healthier Life.* Retrieved from AARP: https://www.aarp.org

Firman, J. a. (2018). *Aging Mastery Playbook.* Arlington, VA: National Council on Aging.

Franke, T. T.-G. (2013). The secrets of higly active older adults. *Journal of Aging Studies, 27(4)*, 398-409.

Friend, T. (2018). *The Chicken Runs at Midnight.* Grand Rapids, MI: Zondervan.

Gerst-Emerson, K. a. (2015, April 8). *Loneliness as a Public Health Issue: The Impact of Loneliness on Health Care Utilization Among Older Adults.* Retrieved from American Journal of Public Health: https://ajph.aphapublications.org

Gray, A. S. (2001, Second Collection). *Lists to Live by.* Sisters, Oregon: Multnomah Publishers, Inc.

Greger, M. a. (2015). *How Not to Die.* New York: Flatiron Books.

Hayes, Kim. (2017). *Friends Can Boost Health, Well-Being Among Older Adults* (Vols. July 6, 2017). AARP.

Hidden in Plain Sight. (2019). Retrieved from University of California–San Francisco, "Sugar Science": http://sugarscience.ucsf.edu/hidden-in-plain-sight/#.XNI2P5NKjs0

Holt-Lunstad, J. R. (2017). Advancing Social Connection as a Public Health Priority in the United States. *American Psychologist, 72*(6), 517-530.

Holy Bible. (2011). In H. Bible, *New International Version (R), NIV(R)* (pp. Also 1973, 1978, 1984). Biblica, Inc. Retrieved from https://www.biblegateway.com/passage/?search=Psalm+23

Howard, J. N. (2002). Legacy [Recorded by N. Nordeman]. On *Woven & Spun.*

Huang, P. L. (2009). A Comprehensive Definition for Metabolic Syndrome. *May-June.*

Hyman, M. (2016). *Eat Fat, Get Thin: Why the Fat we Eat is the Key to Sustained Weight Loss and Vibrant Health.* New York: Little, Brown Spark.

Ingram, J. H. (2018). Well Done [Recorded by T. Afters]. On *The Beginning & Everything After.* Nashville (2018), TN: F. Trade.

Johnston, R. (2014). *The Hope Quotient: Measure It. Raise It. You'll Never Be the Same.* Nashville, TN: Thomas Nelson Publishing.

Joseph, S. (2013). *What Doesn't Kill Us: The New Psychology of Posttraumatic Growth.* New York: Basic Books.

Kay, D. (2015). *Note to Self–Daily Reminders for the Brokenhearted.* Retrieved from Hope for the Broken Hearted Ministries: https://notetoselfdailyremindersforthebrokenhearted.wordpress.com/

Kristeller, J. P. (2015). *The Joy of Half a Cookie: Using Mindfulness to Lose Weight and End the Struggle with Food.* London: Carmelite House, Orion PublishingGroup Ltd.

Lindland E., K.-T. N. (2016). Gauging aging: Expert and public understandings of aging in America. *Communication and the Public*, 211-229.

Little Engine That Could. (2014). Retrieved from National Public Radio: https://www.npr.org/2014/07/08/329520062

Lombardi, V. a. (2006). *What It Takes To Be Number One.* Naperville, Illinois: SimpleTruths, an imprint of Sourcebooks, Inc.

Lundy-Ekman, L. (2007). *Neuroscience: Fundamentals for Rehabilitation.* St. Louis, MO: Saunders/Elsevier.

Maddux, J. S. (2005). *Self-Efficacy: The power of believing you can.* New York: Oxford University Press.

Madell, R. (2016, March 14). *Battling the Stress of Living with Chronic Illness.* Retrieved from Healthline: https://www.healthline.com/health/depression/chronic-illness#1

Mahmud, A. (2017, August 20). *Changing Mindsets.* Retrieved from University of Portsmouth: http://mindsets.port.ac.uk/?p=80

Martens, A., Johns, M., Greenberg, J., & Schimel, J. (2006). Combating stereotype threats: The effect of self-affirmation on women's intellectual performance. *Journal of Experimental Social Psychology*, 236-243.

Maxwell, J. C. (2005). *25 Ways to Win With People.* Nashville, Tennessee: Thomas Nelson, Inc.

Mayo Clinic. (2016, September 28). *Adult Health.* Retrieved from Mayo Clinic: https://www.mayoclinic.org/healthy-lifestyle/adult-health/in-depth/friendships/art-20044860

Miller, J. (2020). *Productivity*. Retrieved from The Muse: https://www.themuse.com/advice/the-secret-to-better-work-manage-your-energy-not-your-time

Mouton, C., Rodabough, R., Rovi, S., Brzyski, R., & Katerndahl, D. (2010). Psychosocial Effects of Physical and Verbal Abuse in Postmenopausal Women. *Annals of Family Medicine*, 206-213.

Mullen, S. M. (2012). Physical Activity and Functional Limitations in Older Adults: The Influence of Self-Efficacy and Functional Performance. *Journals of Gerontology, Series B, Volume 67B*(3), 354-361.

Neff, K. P. (2015). *Self-Compassion: The Proven Power of Being Kind to Yourself*. William Morrow.

North, M. (2015). Ageism Stakes Its Claim in the Social Sciences. *Generations*, 29.

Ogle, S. (2014, January 13). *My Best Secret for Killing Procrastination and Getting Stuff Done*. Retrieved from Location Rebel: https://www.locationrebel.com/getting-stuff-done/

Ouchida, K. a. (2015). Not for Doctors Only: Ageism in Healthcare. *Generations*, 46.

Oxford Dictionary of English. (2015). Dictionary. Oxford: Oxford University Press. Retrieved from http://www.oxfordreference.com/

Peppler, M. (2013, July 5). Top 5 Ways to Get Your Goddess On! *Smart Healthy Women: Because You Matter*.

Piper, W. (1957). *The Little Engine That Could*. Platt & Munk.

Piscatella, J. C. (2010). *Positive Mind, Healthy Heart*. New York: Workman Publishing.

Playforth, C. (2019, July 12). *How to Do Mind Checks with Philippians 4:8*. Retrieved from Arabah Joy: ArabahJoy.com

PositivePsychology.org.uk. (2008). What is Self-Efficacy? Bandura's Four Sources of Efficacy Beliefs. *PositivePsychology.org.uk*. Retrieved from http://positivepsychology.org.uk/self-efficacy-definition-bandura-meaning/

Puff, R. (2017, June 4). *Bad Things Happen to Everyone*. Retrieved from Psychology Today: https://www.psychologytoday.com/us/blog/meditation-modern-life/201706/bad-things-happen-everyone

Qualls, S. (2014). What Social Relationships can do for Health. *Generations*, 8-14.

Relationships, Health, and Well-Being Later in Life. (2014, Spring). *Generations*. San Francisco, CA: Joural of the American Society on Aging.

Rigsby, S. a. (2009). *Unthinkable.* Carol Stream, IL: Tyndale House Publishers, Inc.

Robbins. (2015). Gauging Aging: How Does the American Public Truly Perceive Older Age and Older People? *Generations*.

Robbins, L. (2015). Combating Ageism with the Power of Knowledge–and a New (Reframed) Perspective. *Generations*.

Roth, E. (Writer), & Fincher, D. (Director). (2008). *The Curious Case of Benjamin Button* [Motion Picture].

Sallis, J. F. (2015). *Physical Activity: Numerous Benefits and Effective Interventions.* Retrieved from Agency for Healthcare Research and Quality: http://www.ahrq.gov/professionals/education/curriculum-tools/population-health/sallis.html

Saturday Night Live. (n.d.). *http://snltranscripts.jt.org/91/91asmalley.phtml*.

Schmidt, G. (2020, May 8). *A Diploma Six Decades in the Making.* Retrieved from USC News: news.usc.edu

Schulze, H. a. (2018, April 16). Loneliness: An Epidemic? *Harvard University Graduate School of Arts and Sciences Blog*.

Seligman, M. (2006). *Learned Optimism: How to Change Your Mind and Your Life.* New York: Vintage.

Sherman, D. B. (2009). Psychological vulnerability and stress: The effects of self-affirmation on sympathetic nervous system responses to naturalistic stressors. *Health Psychology, 28*, 554-562.

Sinek, S. (2009). *Start With Why.* London: Portfolio Penguin.

Soukup, R. (2019). *Do it Scared.* Grand Rapids, MI: Zondervan.

Thomas, M. (2014). *It Ain't Over... Till It's Over.* New York: Simon & Schuster, Inc.

U.S. Navy. (n.d.). *Navy Seals.* Retrieved from Navy Seals Training Stages: www.sealswcc.com/navy-seal-training-stages.html

UK Phrase Finder. (n.d.). *http://www.phrases.org.uk/meanings/you-cant-teach-an-old-dog-new-tricks.html.*

VIA Institute on Character Strengths . (n.d.). Retrieved from https://www.viacharacter.org/

Wallace, P., McKinlay, B., Coletta, N., Vlaar, J., Taber, M., Wilson, P., & Cheung, S. (2017). Effects of Motivational Self-Talk on Endurance and Cognitive Performance in the Heat. *American College of Sports Medicine.*

Wax, E., Zieve, D., & Conaway, B. (2018, July 14). *Portion Size.* Retrieved from MedlinePlus: https://medlineplus.gov/ency/patientinstructions/000337.htm

Webb, C. (2016). *How to Have a Good Day.* New York: Crown Publishing Group.

Westerhoff, N. (December 2008). Set in Our Ways: Why Change is So Hard. *Scientific American.* Retrieved from https://www.scientificamerican.com/magazine/mind/2008/12-01/

Wichmann, S. (2017, July). *The Little Engine That Could.* Retrieved from Virginia Reperatory Theater: http://va-rep.org/z_the-little-engine-that-could-childrens-theatre-willow-lawn.html

Woodward, N. W. (1987). Age and health care beliefs: Self-efficacy as a mediator of low desire for control. *Psychol. Aging.*

Table of Affirmations

Figure 1	*Amaging*™ Affirmation Outline	20
Figure 2	*Amaging*™ Affirmation to Do the Write Thing!	25
Figure 3	*Amaging*™ Affirmation: Be More Positive about Growing Older	47
Figure 4	*Amaging*™ Affirmation: Building a Habit to Plan My Day	67
Figure 5	*Amaging*™ Affirmation for Self-Compassion	76
Figure 6	*Amaging*™ Affirmation to Rise and Shine!	87
Figure 7	*Amaging*™ Affirmation on Friendship	102
Figure 8	*Amaging*™ Affirmation to Move More	109
Figure 9	Elasticity for the Soul: Resourcefulness Affirmation	113
Figure 10	Stuck on Savory *Amaging*™ Affirmation	124
Figure 11	*Amaging*™ Affirmation to Pray More	138
Figure 12	New Habit Affirmation	154
Figure 13	*Amaging*™ Affirmation on Achieving Goals	160

Made in the USA
Middletown, DE
20 November 2022

15618189R00104